The Everyday HEART HEALTHY COOKBOOK for Beginners

by Ruby Larson

Contents

Chapter 7: Snacks & Side Recipes - Healthy Bites Throughout the Day

Chapter 8: Soup & Stew Recipes

Chapter 9: Poultry and Meat Recipes

Chapter 10: Seafood and Fish Recipes

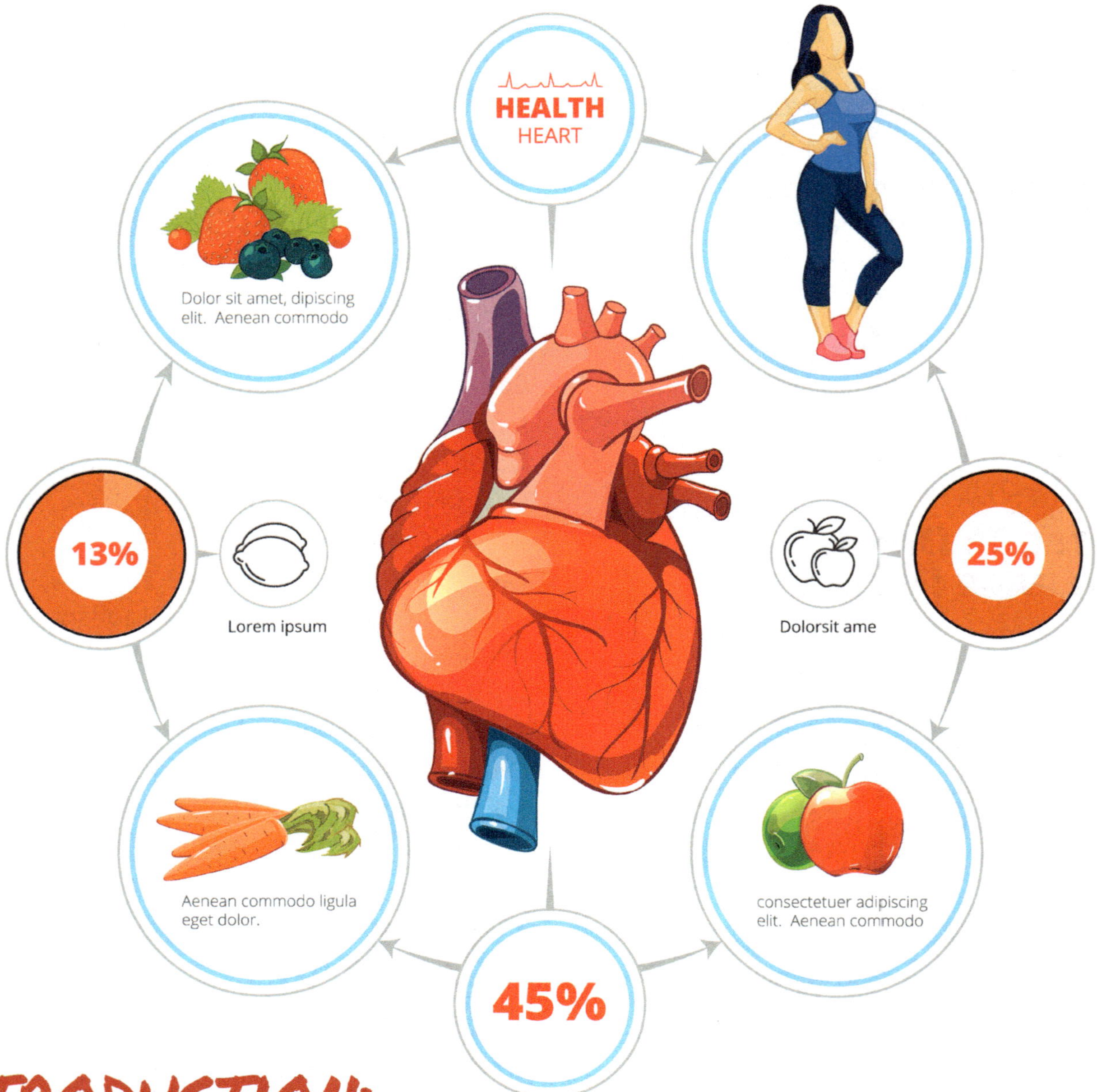

INTRODUCTION: SETTING THE STAGE FOR A HEART-HEALTHY LIFESTYLE

Welcome to «The Everyday Heart Healthy Cookbook for Beginners.» I'm D. Rose, thrilled to guide you toward a healthier heart. In this Introduction, we'll set the stage for your transformation into a heart-conscious culinary artist, covering every vital point to pave the way for a heart-healthy lifestyle.

The Power of Food for Heart Health:

Your Heart is the engine that powers your body, and what you eat has a profound impact on its performance. A heart-healthy diet can help you control your blood pressure, lower your cholesterol, and minimize your chance of developing heart disease. It's about what you avoid and embracing the nourishing foods that fortify your Heart.

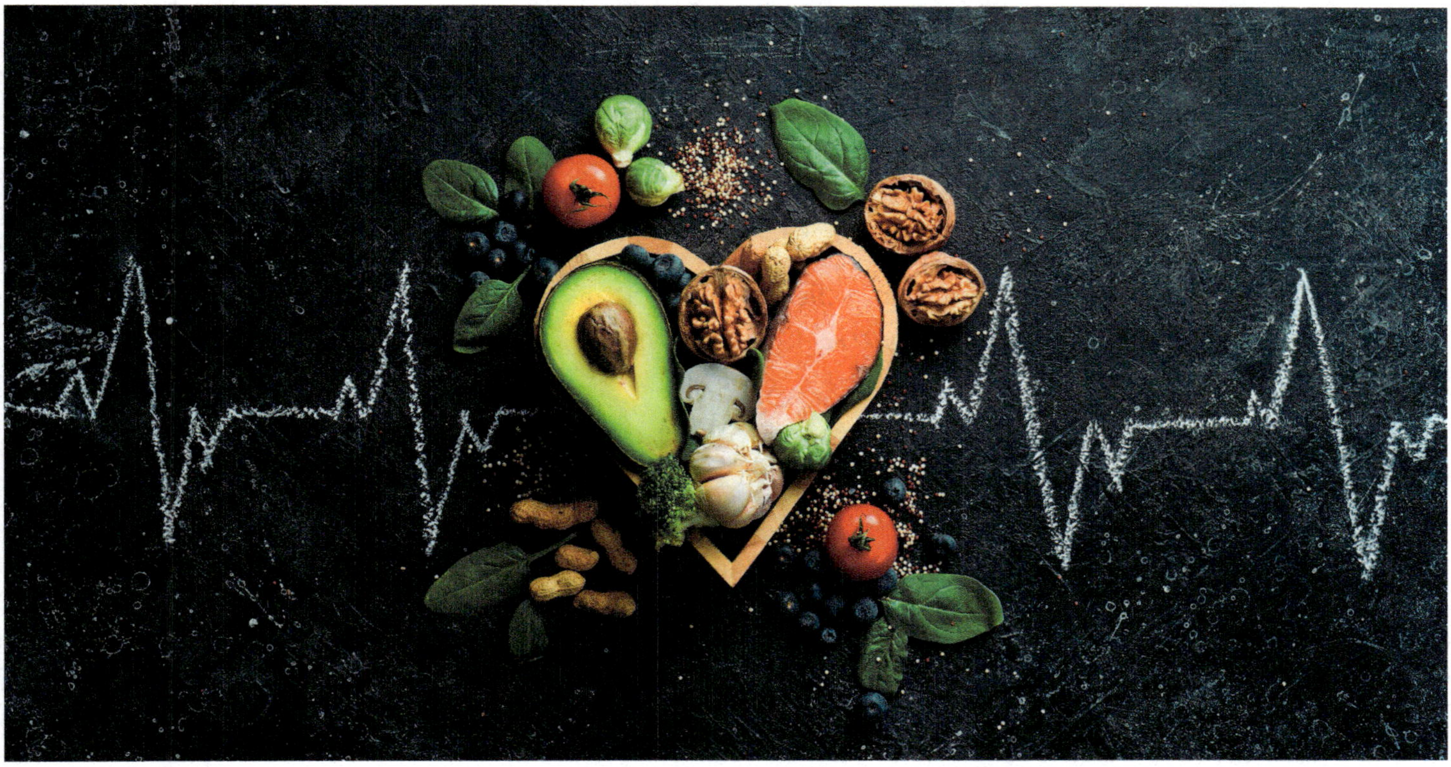

The Beginner's Advantage:

If you're new to the world of heart-healthy eating, consider yourself fortunate. As a beginner, you have a clean slate to work with, unburdened by old habits. You'll discover that adopting a heart-healthy diet can be an exciting adventure filled with new flavors and health benefits.

Making Heart Health Accessible:

One of the core principles of this cookbook is accessibility. I've crafted these recipes with beginners in mind, ensuring that each dish is easy to prepare and bursting with heart-healthy goodness. You only need to be willing to put your Heart's health first; you don't need to be a chef or have a cupboard stocked with exotic items.

Building a Foundation:

Building a heart-healthy lifestyle requires a strong foundation. In this cookbook, you'll find delicious recipes and valuable knowledge. We'll explore the basics of a heart-healthy diet, covering essential topics like understanding dietary needs, managing sodium, fats, and cholesterol, and mastering portion control.

The Role of Knowledge:

Knowledge is your most potent tool on this journey. By understanding the science behind heart-healthy eating, you'll make informed choices that empower your Heart. You'll learn how to navigate food labels, decipher between good and bad fats, and uncover the secrets of portion control.

Beyond diet:

While nutrition is pivotal in heart health, it's not the only aspect to consider. We'll discuss the importance of physical activity, stress management, and overall well-being. A holistic approach to health enhances the benefits of a heart-healthy diet.

The Joy of Cooking:

Cooking should never be a chore; it should be a joy. I want you to savor the experience of preparing heart-healthy meals. You'll discover that with a few culinary tricks and techniques, you can turn fresh, wholesome ingredients into delectable dishes that nourish your Heart and soul.

A Sustainable Lifestyle:

Sustainability is key. This is not a crash diet; it's a lifestyle shift. We'll explore how to integrate heart-healthy eating into your daily routine, making it a sustainable, lifelong practice.

A Community of Support:

You're not alone on this journey. Whether it's the community of fellow beginners, your family, or friends, having a support system can make all the difference. Share your goals, experiences, and triumphs with others—a powerful motivator.

Your Heart, Your Future:

Remember, the heart-healthy lifestyle you will embrace is an investment in your future. It's a gift to yourself and your loved ones. As we embark on this culinary adventure together, remember your incredible potential to improve your Heart's health and enhance your overall quality of life.

I'm excited to be your companion as we explore the delicious world of heart-healthy cooking. Together, we'll make each meal a testament to your love and care for your Heart. Let's begin this transformative journey towards a healthier, happier you.

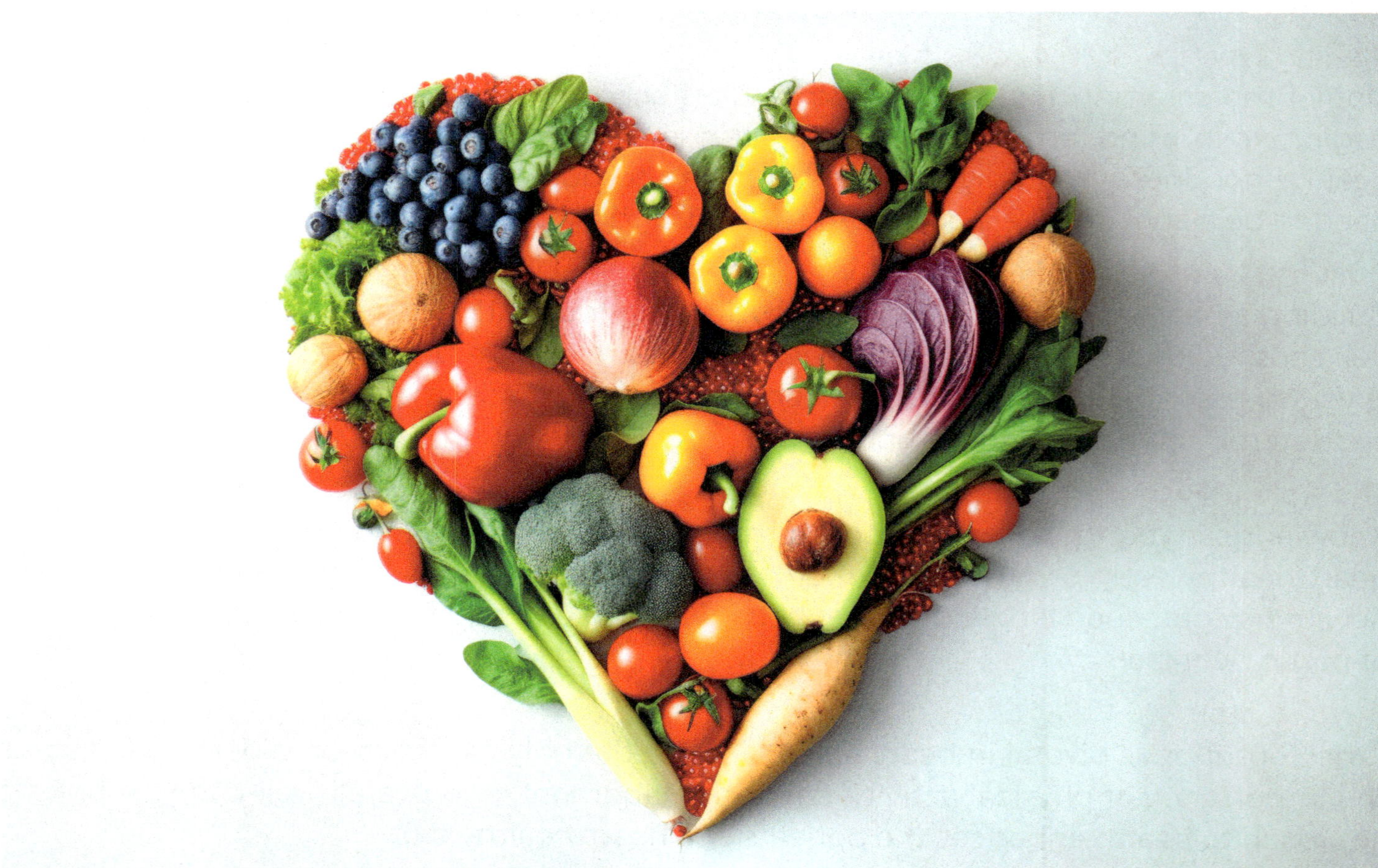

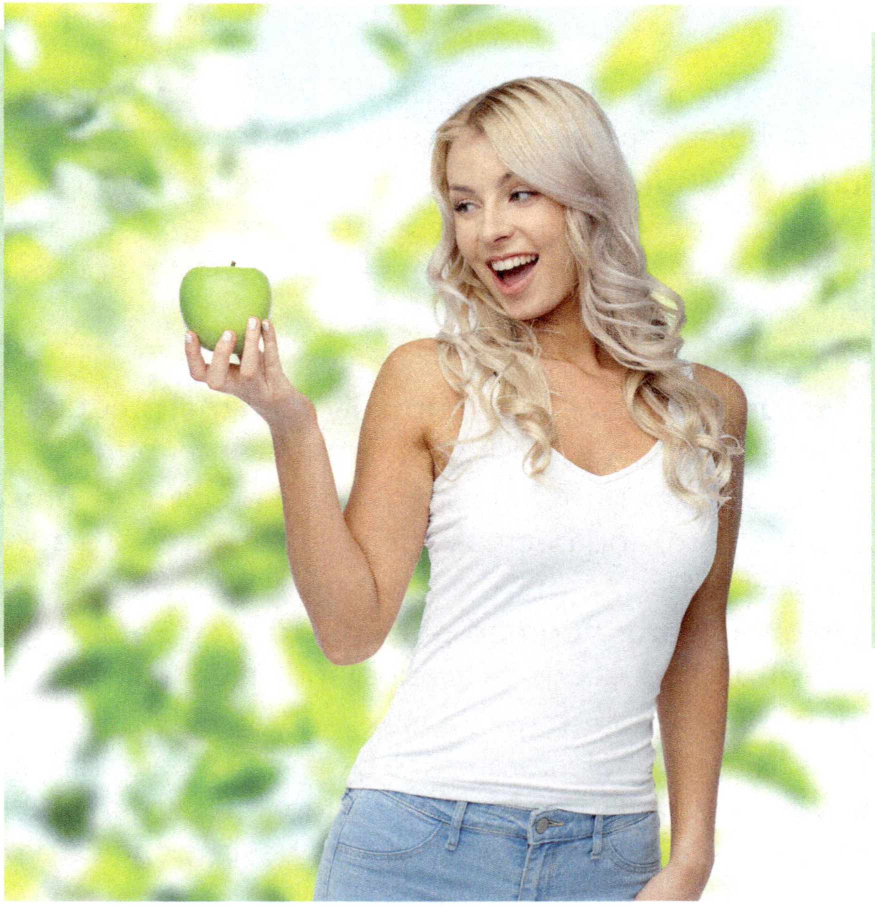

The Basic Principles of the Heart-Healthy Diet

Understanding Dietary Needs & Nutritional Balance

To truly embrace a heart-healthy diet, we must first understand our dietary needs and the balance of nutrients our bodies require to function optimally.

- **Macronutrients:** The nutrients our body needs in more significant amounts: carbohydrates, proteins, and fats. Each plays a specific role. Carbohydrates provide Energy, proteins are essential for repair and growth, and fats support cell function and Energy.
    - **Carbohydrates:** Choose complex carbohydrates over simple sugars and refined grains, such as whole grains, vegetables, and fruits.
    - **Proteins:** Choose lean protein sources such as poultry, fish, beans, and legumes. Limit red meat and select cuts that are lower in fat.
    - **Fats:** It's essential to differentiate between unhealthy fats (saturated and trans fats) and heart-healthy fats (monounsaturated and polyunsaturated fats).
- **Micronutrients** include vitamins and minerals, necessary in smaller amounts but equally vital. They aid in energy production, bone maintenance, immune function, and more.
- **Water:** The most overlooked yet crucial component. It aids digestion, hydration, and nutrient transportation.
- **Fiber:** Crucial for digestive health and also beneficial for heart health; aim to incorporate whole grains, fruits, vegetables, and legumes into your diet.

The Role of Sodium, Fats, & Cholesterol in Heart Health

Diet plays a pivotal role in heart health. When consumed in inappropriate amounts, sodium, fats, and cholesterol can become risk factors for heart-related ailments.

- **Sodium:** For the maintenance of fluid balance and neuronal function, sodium is crucial. However, consuming too much sodium can increase blood pressure, a risk factor for heart disease. Limiting processed foods and being mindful of salt in cooking can help manage sodium intake.
- **Fats:** Not all fats are created equal.
  - **Saturated Fats:** Found primarily in animal products, these can raise blood cholesterol levels. Limit by choosing lean meats and opting for low-fat dairy products.
  - **Trans Fats:** Trans fats, frequently present in processed meals, can increase bad cholesterol and decrease good cholesterol. It's advisable to avoid these as much as possible.
  - **Monounsaturated and polyunsaturated Fats:** These are heart-friendly fats. Sources include nuts, seeds, avocados, and certain oils like olive oil.
- **Cholesterol:** Cholesterol is a waxy substance produced by the liver and found in certain foods. Dietary cholesterol, once believed to be a significant factor in blood cholesterol, is now understood to have a more minor effect than previously thought. It's crucial to limit saturated and trans fats to maintain healthy cholesterol levels.

Portion Control: Quantity vs. Quality

While choosing the right foods is essential, how much you eat is equally crucial.

Understanding Portions: With the rise of super-sized meals, our understanding of standard portions has become skewed. Familiarize yourself with serving sizes. For instance, a plate of beef should resemble a deck of cards in size.

- **Mindful Eating:** Pay attention to your body's hunger and fullness cues. Eat slowly, savor each bite, and learn to recognize when you're comfortably full.
- **Balanced Plate:** Visual cues can be helpful. Aim for a plate half filled with vegetables, a quarter with lean protein, and a quarter with whole grains.
- **Quality Over Quantity:** Always prioritize the quality of the food you consume. Nutrient-dense foods like vegetables, fruits, lean proteins, and whole grains nourish your body more than calorie-dense, nutrient-poor foods.

In conclusion, embracing a heart-healthy diet is not about deprivation but about making informed, balanced choices. As we journey further into this book, we'll explore how to translate these principles into delicious, heart-healthy meals that cater to all tastes and preferences.

Stay passionate about your Heart's health. It begins a journey filled with delicious discoveries and transformative choices.

Benefits of a Heart-Healthy Diet

A heart-healthy diet is more than a mere approach to eating; it's an investment in your future and a pledge to honor the organ that tirelessly powers your every moment. This chapter seeks to illuminate the myriad benefits of a heart-healthy lifestyle, from the obvious to the subtle, all-bearing testament to the transformative power of mindful eating.

Longer, More Vibrant Life

A profound promise lies at the core of a heart-healthy diet: the potential for a lengthened life but one bursting with vibrancy and vigor.

- **Disease Prevention:** A diet that supports heart health actively works against the leading causes of morbidity and mortality worldwide, such as coronary artery disease, strokes, and heart attacks. By making heart-conscious choices, you're bolstering your defenses against these ailments.
- **Organ Health:** While the Heart is the central beneficiary, other organs thrive in a heart-healthy environment. The liver, kidneys, and brain benefit from reduced saturated fats, controlled sodium levels, and an increased intake of antioxidants.
- **Aging Gracefully:** Nutrient-rich, heart-healthy diets can slow down the natural wear and tear, leading to healthier skin, stronger bones, and reduced age-related diseases.

Improved Blood Pressure & Cholesterol Levels

The blood coursing through our veins and arteries is the lifeline of every cell, and its health is intrinsically tied to blood pressure and cholesterol.

- **Balanced Blood Pressure:** Excessive sodium and low potassium intake can cause high blood pressure (hypertension), a silent killer. A heart-healthy diet emphasizes reduced sodium and increased potassium, leading to balanced blood pressure levels.
- **Optimal Cholesterol:** By minimizing the intake of trans fats and saturated fats, the heart-healthy diet ensures a reduction in LDL (bad cholesterol) levels. Including omega-3 fatty acids from sources like fish aids in increasing HDL (good cholesterol) levels.
- **Vascular Health:** Improved blood pressure and cholesterol levels ensure that blood vessels remain elastic and unblocked. This is essential to prevent conditions like arteriosclerosis.

Enhanced Energy and overall Well-being

Beyond the metrics of blood pressure and cholesterol lies a realm of benefits that, while less tangible, significantly impact daily life.

- **Consistent Energy Levels:** The emphasis on whole grains, lean proteins, and healthy fats in the heart-healthy diet guarantees a constant release of Energy, preventing the highs and lows linked to diets high in sugar.

- **Mood Regulation:** Foods rich in omega-3 fatty acids, like walnuts and fatty fish, are linked to reduced risks of depression and mood disorders. Furthermore, stable blood sugar levels from a balanced diet can prevent mood swings.
- **Digestive Harmony:** Focusing on fiber-rich foods aids in smooth digestion and regular bowel movements, preventing constipation, bloating, and other gastrointestinal problems.
- **Enhanced Sleep Patterns:** A balanced diet can regulate blood sugar levels, ensuring more profound and restful sleep and rejuvenated mornings and productive days.

A heart-healthy diet is the cornerstone of a life lived fully and joyfully. Its benefits cascade into every facet of existence, reminding us that the choices we make at the dining table reverberate far beyond the confines of the kitchen. As we delve deeper into this book, you'll find that each recipe, tip, and suggestion celebrates this life-affirming philosophy.

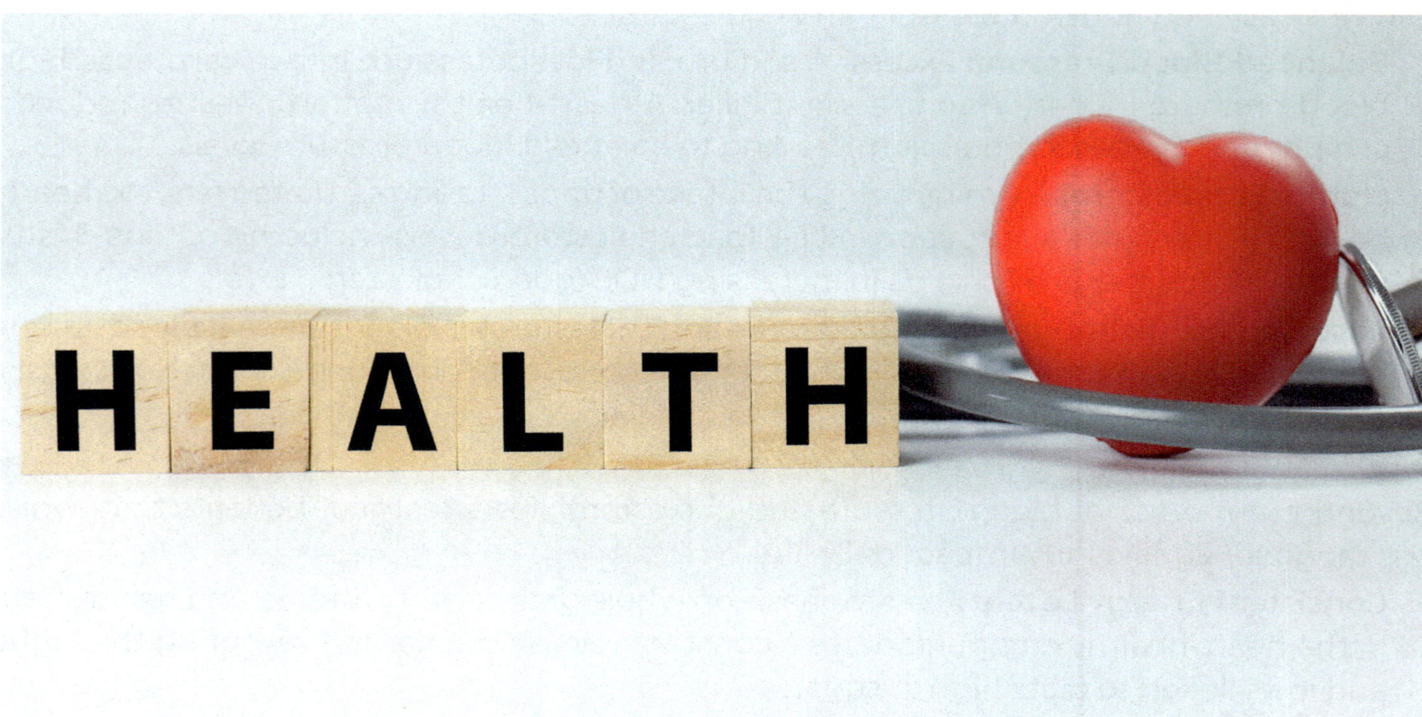

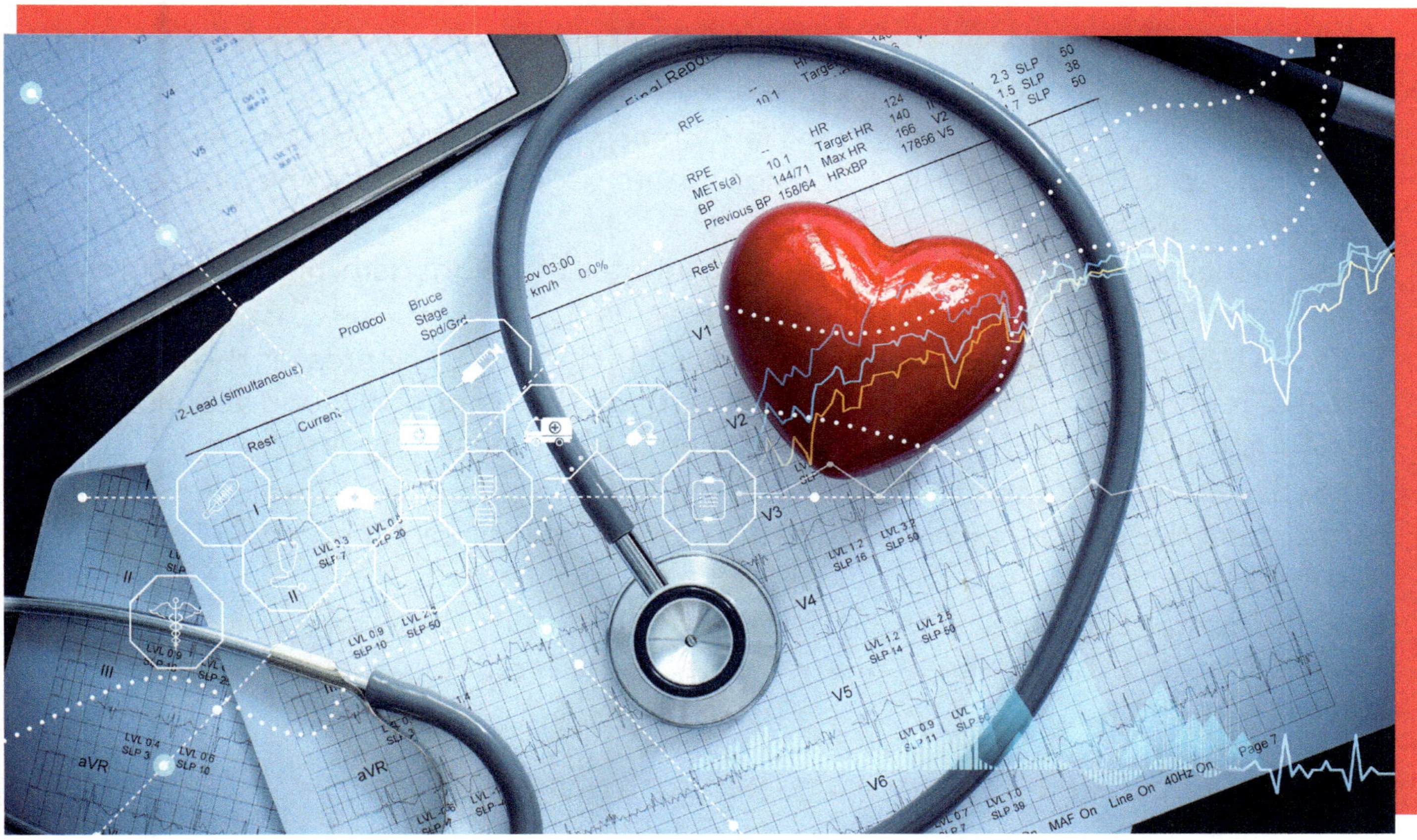

What Are the Risk Factors for Heart Disease?

Heart disease often deemed the «silent killer», manifests through various risk factors. Some risk factors are beyond our control, while others can be managed or even reversed through lifestyle changes. Recognizing and understanding these factors is pivotal in shaping our health choices and, thus, the trajectory of our heart health. Let's delve into these risk factors and dissect their implications.

Genetic Predispositions

Our genes, inherited from our ancestors, play a significant role in determining various health outcomes, including our susceptibility to heart disease.

- **Family History:** Your risk is higher if an immediate family member (like a parent or sibling) has had heart disease, especially at a young age. This familial trend suggests a genetic component.
- **Ethnicity:** Certain ethnic groups, notably African and South Asian populations, have shown a heightened risk of heart disease. These predispositions could be due to genetics, lifestyle, and environmental factors.
- **Genetic Disorders:** Some rare genetic disorders, such as familial hypercholesterolemia, directly impact heart health by causing elevated cholesterol levels from a young age. While genetic predispositions cannot be altered, awareness allows for early interventions and preventive measures, making a significant difference in outcomes.

Lifestyle Choices & Environmental Factors

Our daily choices and the environment we reside in profoundly influence heart health.

- **Diet:** Diets high in saturated fats, trans fats, cholesterol, and sodium can elevate the risk of heart disease. Conversely, diets lacking in fruits, vegetables, and whole grains miss out on heart-protective benefits.
- **Physical Inactivity:** A sedentary lifestyle contributes to weight gain, high blood pressure, and poor circulation, all elevating heart disease risks.
- **Tobacco Use:** Smoking or using tobacco products significantly increases the risk of heart disease. Tobacco harmful substances can damage the heart and blood vessels, leading to plaque buildup (atherosclerosis), which can result in heart attacks.
- **Excessive Alcohol Consumption:** While moderate alcohol consumption might have some protective effects, excessive drinking can lead to high blood pressure, heart failure, and strokes.
- **Environmental Stressors:** Chronic stress, whether from work, relationships, or other sources, can contribute to heart disease, especially if it leads to poor habits like unhealthy eating or smoking.

Previous Medical History & its Implications

Past medical conditions can provide crucial insights into one's vulnerability to heart disease.

- **High Blood Pressure:** Chronic hypertension strains the Heart, damages arteries, and increases the risk of heart attack, stroke, and heart failure.
- **High Cholesterol:** Elevated LDL cholesterol levels can lead to atherosclerosis, reducing blood flow and increasing the risk of a heart attack.
- **Diabetes:** Heart disease is more common in people with diabetes, mainly if blood sugar levels aren't well-controlled. High blood sugar levels can harm the Heart's nerves and blood vessels.
- **Previous Cardiovascular Events:** Those who've had heart attacks or strokes in the past are more susceptible to future events.
- **Rheumatic Heart Disease, Congenital Heart Defects:** Conditions that have directly affected the heart structure or function in the past can have lasting implications, necessitating lifelong monitoring and care.

A thorough understanding of the risk factors for heart disease provides a clear picture that allows people to take targeted action. While some factors, like genetics, remain unmodifiable, many risk elements rooted in lifestyle and previous health history can be addressed. The subsequent chapters will guide you in navigating these modifiable risks through diet, equipping you with the tools to champion your Heart's health.

A List of Foods to Eat, Limit, and Avoid

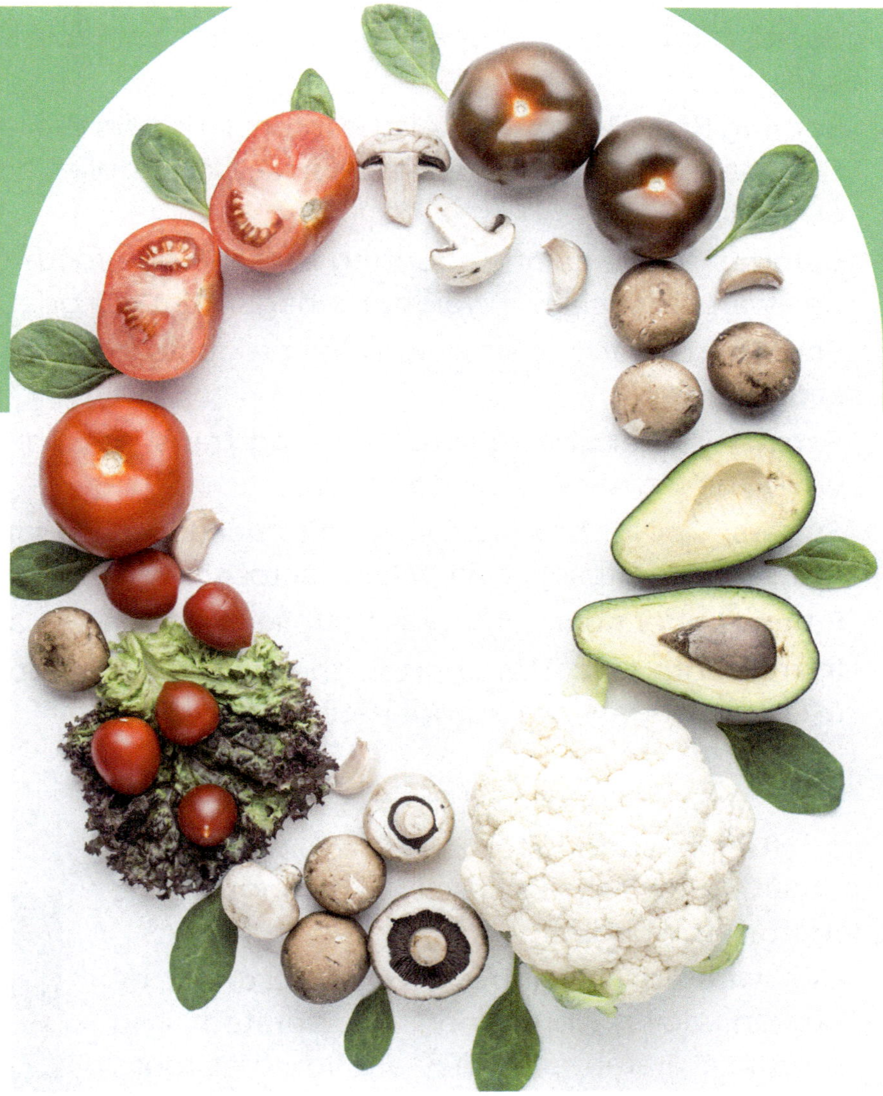

For heart-conscious individuals, navigating the vast sea of available foods can feel overwhelming. However, understanding the nuances of nutrition and embracing the heart-healthy pantry can transform this journey into a delightful culinary adventure. This chapter guides you through the essentials, helps you decode the enigma of food labels, and demystifies fats.

The Heart-Healthy Pantry: Staple Items for Your Kitchen

A well-stocked kitchen is the cornerstone of a heart-healthy diet. Here are the staples you should always have on hand:

- **Whole Grains:** Quinoa, brown rice, barley, oatmeal, whole grain bread and pasta.
- **Lean Proteins:** Poultry, fish (especially fatty fish like salmon, mackerel, and sardines), tofu, legumes, and beans.
- **Healthy Fats:** Olive oil, avocado, nuts (like almonds and walnuts), and seeds (like chia and flaxseed).
- **Vegetables:** A colorful variety, including leafy greens, bell peppers, carrots, and broccoli.
- **Fruits:** Berries, apples, bananas, citrus fruits, and more.
- **Dairy & Alternatives:** Low-fat or non-fat yogurt, milk, or plant-based alternatives like almond or soy milk.
- **Herbs & Spices:** Basil, rosemary, turmeric, black pepper, and garlic — nature's way of adding flavor without excess salt!
- **Beverages:** Water, herbal teas, and moderate amounts of coffee.

Decoding Food Labels: What to Watch Out For

Understanding food labels can equip you with valuable information. Here's what you should look for:

- **Serving Size:** Begin here. All the information on the label applies to this specific amount. Beware of products where the packaging implies a single serving, but the label states otherwise.
- **Calories:** While calorie counting isn't the sole focus of a heart-healthy diet, it's good to be aware, especially if weight management is a goal.
- **Sodium:** Lower is better. Aim for products with no more than 140mg of sodium per serving.
- **Fats:** Pay attention to saturated and trans fats. The latter should be avoided entirely, while the former should be limited.
- **Sugars:** Opt for products with minimal added sugars. Remember, natural sugars from fruits (like fructose) or dairy (like lactose) are less concerning than added sugars.
- **Fiber:** Higher fiber content is beneficial for heart health.
- **Ingredients List:** The shorter, the better. Avoid products with unfamiliar chemicals, excessive sugars, or hydrogenated oils.

The Truth about Fats: Good vs. Bad

Fats, often misunderstood, play pivotal roles in our health. However, it's crucial to distinguish the good from the bad:

- **Unsaturated Fats (The Good):** These can be broken down into monounsaturated and polyunsaturated fats. They are liquid at room temperature.
- **Sources:** Olive oil, nuts, seeds, and fish.
- **Benefits:** It can help reduce harmful cholesterol levels and provide essential fatty acids.
- **Saturated Fats (Limit):** While not entirely «bad,» these should be consumed in moderation.
- **Sources:** Animal products like beef, butter, cheese, and plant oils like olive oil.
- **Implications:** Can raise total and LDL (bad) cholesterol levels, increasing heart disease risk.
- **Trans Fats (The Bad):** These should be avoided.
- **Sources:** Primarily in processed foods as partially hydrogenated oils.
- **Implications:** Raise lousy cholesterol while lowering good cholesterol, amplifying heart disease risk.

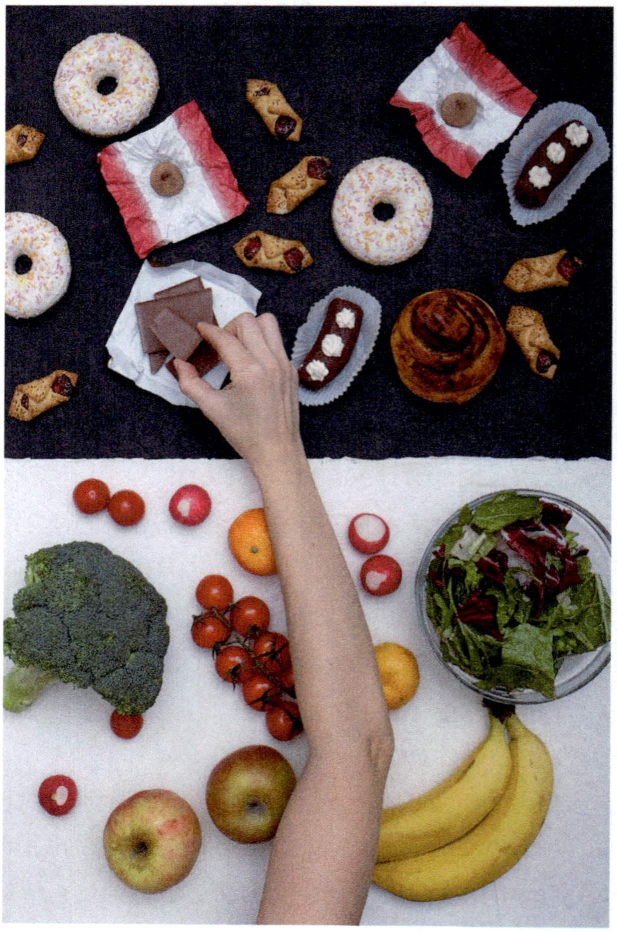

With this knowledge, you can make heart-conscious choices at the grocery store, ensuring your kitchen becomes a sanctuary for heart-healthy foods. As we move forward, we'll explore how to turn these ingredients into delicious, heart-nourishing meals.
Below is a list of products that are notably high in cholesterol, sodium, and fats (table)

Products with High Levels of Sodium:

- **Table Salt:** The primary source of sodium in many diets.
- **Processed Meats:** Such as bacon, ham, salami, and hot dogs.
- **Canned Soups:** Even those labeled «reduced sodium» can still be high in salt.
- **Fast Foods:** Especially fries, burgers, and other fried items.
- **Frozen Dinners:** They often contain large amounts of sodium to enhance flavor and act as a preservative.
- **Processed Snacks:** Such as chips, pretzels, and salted nuts.
- **Pickles and Other Pickled Foods:** Due to the brining process.
- **Soy Sauce:** Even the «reduced-sodium» version can be very high in salt.
- **Canned Vegetables and Beans:** Always check the label; they can be packed with added salt.

Products with High Levels Fats:

- **Butter:** A dairy product that contains a high percentage of saturated fat.
- **Lard:** Rendered pig fat is often used in baking and frying.
- **Shortening:** Commonly used in baking, hydrogenated vegetable oil is high in trans fats.
- **Very Fried Foods**, Such as fried doughnuts and french fries.
- **Processed Snack Foods:** Chips, cookies, and some microwave popcorn varieties.
- **Cream and Cream-Based Products:** Like full-fat ice cream and whipped cream.
- **Processed Meats:** Including sausages, bacon, and salami.
- **Cheese:** Particularly processed cheeses and those that are full-fat.
- **Pastries and Desserts:** Many are made with butter, shortening, and other high-fat ingredients.

For a heart-healthy diet, it's essential to monitor the intake of these products or seek out low-sodium and low-cholesterol alternatives. Always read labels and make informed decisions about the foods you consume.

ALERT

While these recommendations are broadly applicable, individual requirements can differ due to unique health circumstances. To tailor your diet for optimal heart health and nutritional guidance, please seek advice from your physician or registered dietitian.
In the subsequent chapters, you'll find recipes meticulously crafted for heart-healthy eating.
Nutritional details are given for a single portion, except where mentioned differently.

Time to Prepare

Cooking Duration

Number of Servings

Wholesome Smoothies + Juices

MORNING BERRY BLISS SMOOTHIE

Calories: 140 kCal | Protein: 5 g | Carbohydrates: 28 g | Sugar: 18 g | Fat: 2 g | Fiber: 6 g | Cholesterol: 0 mg | Sodium: 60 mg | Phosphorus: 40 mg | Potassium: 350 mg.

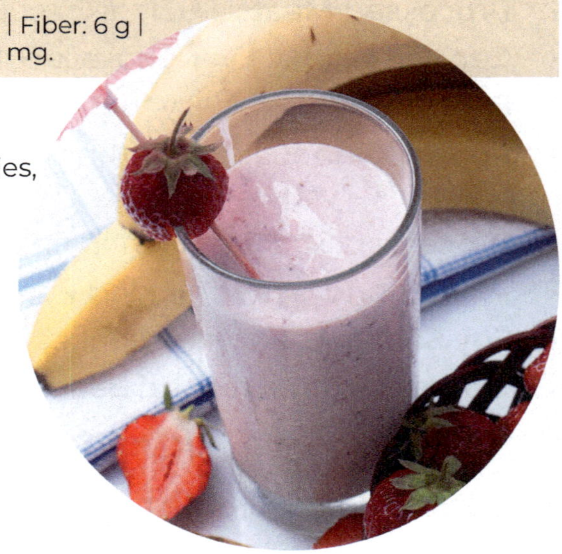

7 min | 0 min | 2

Ingredients:

- 1 cup mixed berries (blueberries, strawberries, raspberries)
- One banana, sliced
- One tablespoon flaxseeds
- 1 cup unsweetened soy milk
- One tablespoon maple syrup (optional)

Directions:

1. In a blender, combine mixed berries, bananas, flaxseeds, and soy milk.
2. Blend until smooth.
3. Add maple syrup if a sweeter taste is desired, and blend for another 10 seconds.
4. Pour into glasses and serve chilled.

Berries are high in antioxidants, which can lower the risk of heart disease, which is why they are heart-healthy. Bananas provide potassium, which is essential for heart health. Flaxseeds have been found to decrease cholesterol levels and contain omega-3 fatty acids beneficial for heart health.

TROPICAL HEART HEALTH DELIGHT

Calories: 160 kCal | Protein: 3 g | Carbohydrates: 30 g | Sugar: 22 g | Fat: 4 g | Fiber: 7 g | Cholesterol: 0 mg | Sodium: 20 mg | Phosphorus: 30 mg | Potassium: 300 mg.

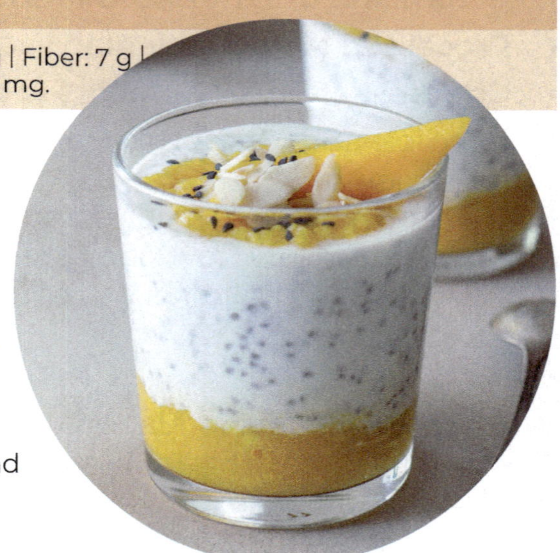

7 min | 0 min | 2

Ingredients:

- 1 cup pineapple chunks
- 1/2 mango, peeled and diced
- 1/2 cup unsweetened coconut milk
- One tablespoon of chia seeds

Directions:

1. In a blender, combine pineapple chunks, mango, coconut milk, and chia seeds.
2. Blend the ingredients at a high speed until the ingredients are well blended at a high speed. The ingredients should be well blended at a high speed. It is smooth.
3. Serve with a pineapple slice around the rim of a tall glass.

Why it's heart-healthy: *Pineapple contains bromelain, an enzyme with anti-inflammatory properties that can benefit heart health. Mangoes are a good source of dietary fiber, vitamins, and minerals, especially potassium, which helps control heart rate and decrease blood pressure. Chia seeds offer omega-3 fatty acids essential for maintaining heart health.*

GINGER PEAR COOLER JUICE

Calories: 95 kCal | Protein: 1 g | Carbohydrates: 25 g | Sugar: 15 g | Fat: 0,5 g | Fiber: 6 g | Cholesterol: 0 mg | Sodium: 5 mg | Phosphorus: 10 mg | Potassium: 220 mg.

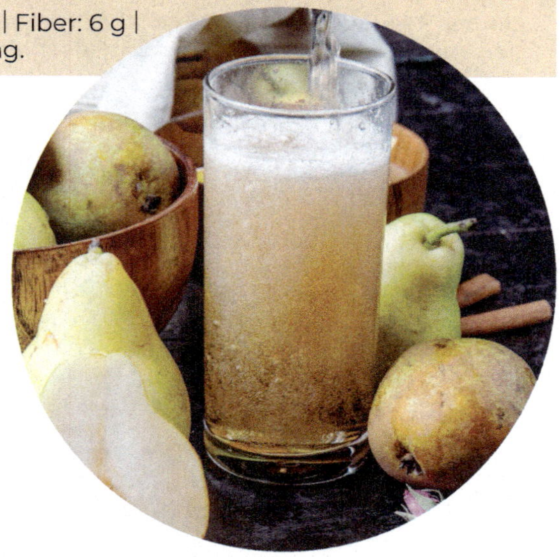

10 min | 0 min | 2

INGREDIENTS:

- Two ripe pears, cored and chopped
- 1-inch ginger, peeled
- 1 cup cold water

DIRECTIONS:

1. In a juicer or blender, combine pears, ginger, and water.
2. Blend or juice until smooth.
3. Pour into glasses and serve chilled.

Heart-Healthy Benefits: *Dietary fiber, which is good for the Heart, may be abundant in pears. Ginger has anti-inflammatory and antioxidative properties.*

RUBY RED GRAPEFRUIT DETOX JUICE

Calories: 95 kCal | Protein: 1 g | Carbohydrates: 23 g | Sugar: 17 g | Fat: 0,2 g | Fiber: 2 g | Cholesterol: 0 mg | Sodium: 10 mg | Phosphorus: 20 mg | Potassium: 250 mg.

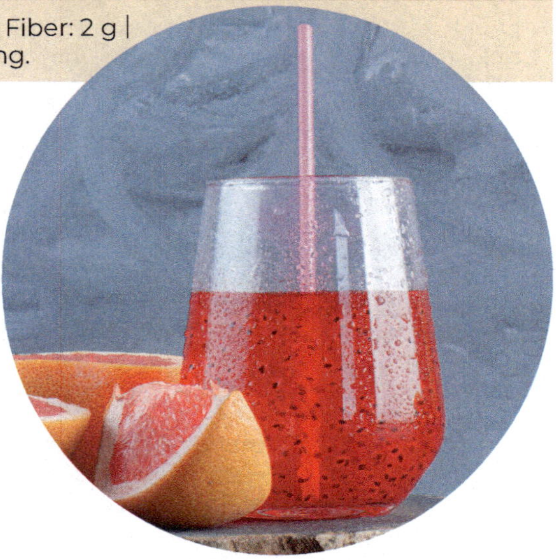

8 min | 0 min | 2

INGREDIENTS:

- Two ruby red grapefruits peeled
- 1 cup cold water
- One tablespoon honey (optional)

DIRECTIONS:

1. In a juicer or blender, combine grapefruits and water.
2. Blend or juice until smooth.
3. Sweeten with honey if desired, mix well, and serve.

Heart-Healthy Benefits: *Vitamin C and antioxidants abound in grapefruits. They help lower bad LDL cholesterol levels and are beneficial for heart health.*

MANGO & STRAWBERRY SUNRISE SMOOTHIE

Calories: 160 kCal | Protein: 2 g | Carbohydrates: 35 g | Sugar: 28 g | Fat: 1 g | Fiber: 4 g | Cholesterol: 0 mg | Sodium: 80 mg | Phosphorus: 30 mg | Potassium: 400 mg.

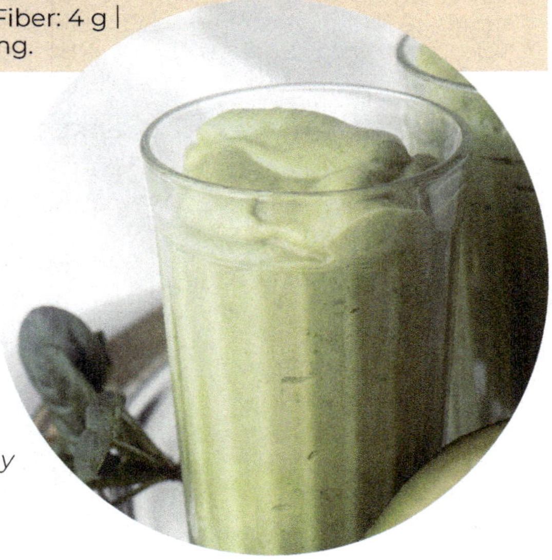

10 min | 0 min | 2

INGREDIENTS:

- One ripe mango, peeled and cubed
- 1 cup fresh strawberries, hulled
- 1 cup almond milk

DIRECTIONS:

1. In a blender, combine mango, strawberries, and almond milk.
2. Blend until smooth and creamy.
3. Pour into glasses and serve immediately.

Heart-Healthy Benefits: *Mangoes contain folate, which can help regulate heart rhythms. Strawberries are known for their heart-healthy antioxidants and polyphenols.*

POMEGRANATE BEET ZINGER JUICE

Calories: 110 kCal | Protein: 2 g | Carbohydrates: 28 g | Sugar: 20 g | Fat: 0,5 g | Fiber: 6 g | Cholesterol: 0 mg | Sodium: 75 mg | Phosphorus: 40 mg | Potassium: 310 mg.

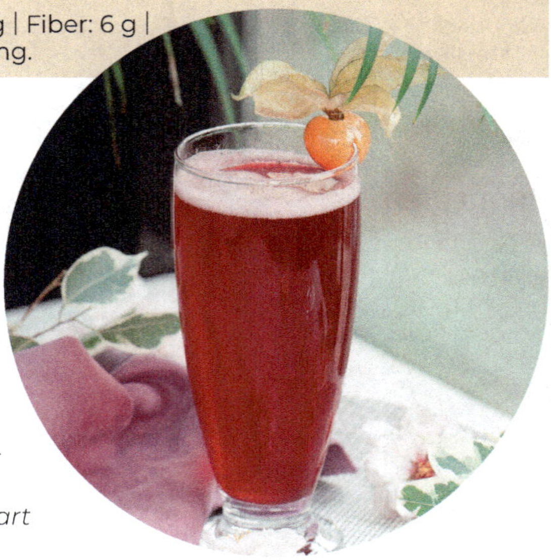

10 min | 0 min | 2

INGREDIENTS:

- One medium beet, peeled and chopped
- 1 cup pomegranate seeds
- One apple, cored and chopped
- 1 cup cold water

DIRECTIONS:

1. In a juicer, combine beet, pomegranate seeds, apple, and water.
2. Blend or juice until smooth.
3. Pour into glasses and serve immediately.

Heart-Healthy Benefits: *Beets and pomegranates are recognized for enhancing blood flow and lowering blood pressure. They're packed with antioxidants and anti-inflammatory properties beneficial for heart health.*

KIWI & SPINACH WAKE-UP SMOOTHIE

Calories: 135 kCal | Protein: 3 g | Carbohydrates: 30 g | Sugar: 18 g | Fat: 1 g | Fiber: 5 g | Cholesterol: 0 mg | Sodium: 55 mg | Phosphorus: 60 mg | Potassium: 540 mg.

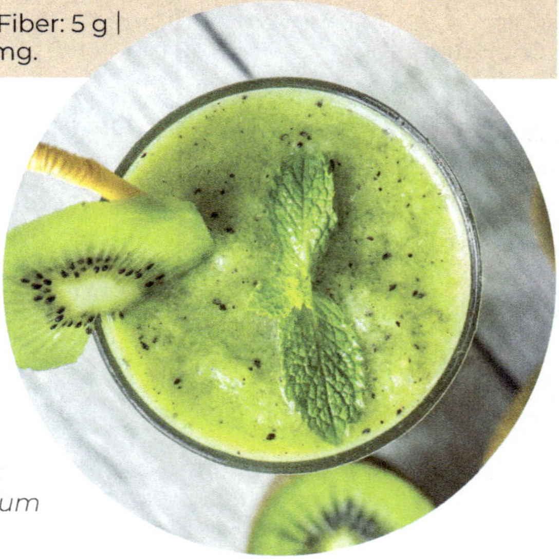

7 min | 0 min | 2

INGREDIENTS:

- Two ripe kiwis, peeled and sliced
- 1 cup fresh spinach leaves
- One banana
- 1 cup almond milk

DIRECTIONS:

1. In a blender, combine the kiwi slices, spinach, banana, and almond milk.
2. Blend until smooth and creamy.
3. Pour into glasses and serve immediately.

Heart-Healthy Benefits: *Kiwi is rich in vitamin C and dietary fiber. Spinach contains lutein, potassium, and folate, all beneficial for heart health. Bananas are an excellent dietary fiber, vitamin C, and potassium source.*

GOLDEN TURMERIC & PINEAPPLE SMOOTHIE

Calories: 160 kCal | Protein: 2 g | Carbohydrates: 22 g | Sugar: 18 g | Fat: 7 g | Fiber: 2 g | Cholesterol: 0 mg | Sodium: 15 mg | Phosphorus: 25 mg | Potassium: 280 mg.

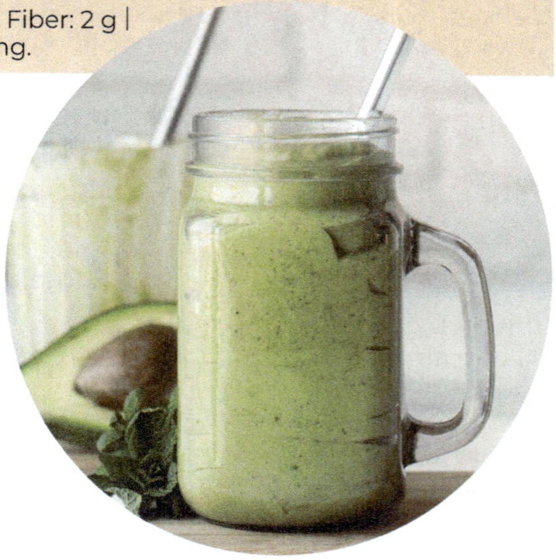

8 min | 0 min | 2

INGREDIENTS:

- 1 cup pineapple chunks
- 1/2 teaspoon turmeric powder
- 1 cup coconut milk
- One tablespoon honey

DIRECTIONS:

1. In a blender, combine the pineapple chunks, turmeric powder, coconut milk, and honey.
2. Blend until smooth.
3. Pour into glasses and serve chilled.

Heart-Healthy Benefits: *Turmeric contains anti-inflammatory curcumin, which can prevent heart diseases. Pineapple provides bromelain, an enzyme known for its anti-inflammatory effects.*

CARROT-ORANGE REVIVE JUICE

Calories: 100 kCal | Protein: 2 g | Carbohydrates: 25 g | Sugar: 15 g | Fat: 0,5 g | Fiber: 5 g | Cholesterol: 0 mg | Sodium: 80 mg | Phosphorus: 45 mg | Potassium: 420 mg.

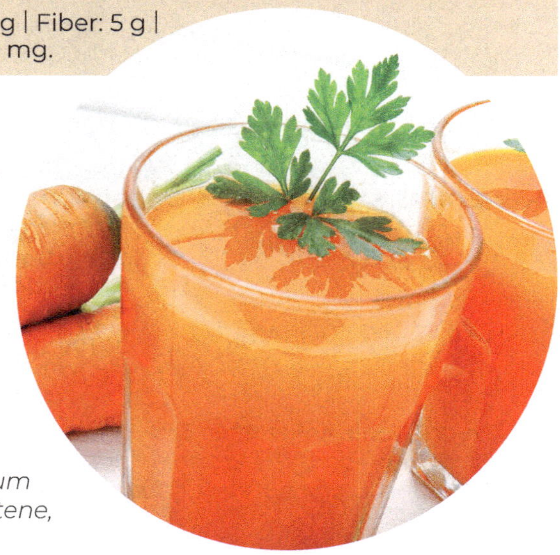

10 min | 0 min | 2

INGREDIENTS:

- Three large carrots, peeled and chopped
- Two oranges, peeled and segmented
- 1-inch piece of ginger, peeled
- 1 cup of cold water

DIRECTIONS:

1. Combine carrots, oranges, ginger, and water in a juicer or blender.
2. Blend or juice until smooth.
3. Pour into glasses and serve immediately.

Heart-Healthy Benefits: *Oranges are high in vitamin C and potassium and are known to maintain heart health. Carrots contain beta-carotene, a powerful antioxidant beneficial for heart health. Ginger has anti-inflammatory properties, which can aid in heart health.*

CREAMY AVOCADO & HONEY SMOOTHIE

Calories: 160 kCal | Protein: 3 g | Carbohydrates: 30 g | Sugar: 22 g | Fat: 4 g | Fiber: 7 g | Cholesterol: 0 mg | Sodium: 20 mg | Phosphorus: 30 mg | Potassium: 300 mg.

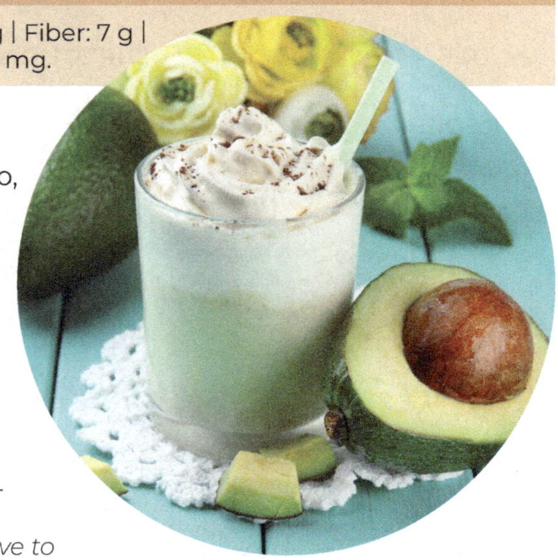

8 min | 0 min | 2

INGREDIENTS:

- One ripe avocado, peeled and pitted
- One tablespoon honey (or to taste)
- 1 cup almond milk
- 1/2 teaspoon vanilla extract

DIRECTIONS:

1. In a blender, combine the avocado, honey, almond milk, and vanilla extract.
2. Blend until smooth and creamy.
3. Taste and adjust sweetness if needed.
4. Pour into glasses and serve chilled.

Heart-Healthy Benefits: *Avocado is rich in monounsaturated, heart-healthy fats. It also provides potassium, which is essential for heart health. Almond milk is a great low-calorie and low-sodium alternative to regular milk.*

NOTES

CRANBERRY ALMOND CRUNCH SMOOTHIE

Calories: 180 kCal | Protein: 4 g | Carbohydrates: 35 g | Sugar: 20 g | Fat: 4 g | Fiber: 5 g | Cholesterol: 0 mg | Sodium: 90 mg | Phosphorus: 70 mg | Potassium: 420 mg.

10 min | 0 min | 2

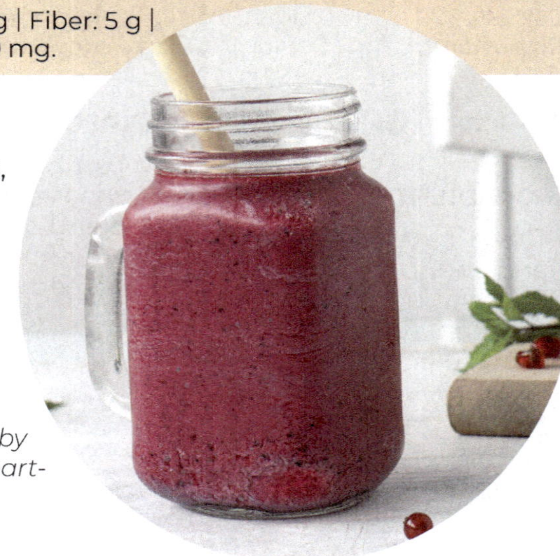

Ingredients:

- 1 cup fresh cranberries
- 10-12 almonds
- One banana
- 1 cup almond milk

Directions:

1. In a blender, combine cranberries, almonds, banana, and almond milk.
2. Blend until creamy and smooth.
3. Pour into glasses and serve chilled.

Heart-Healthy Benefits: *Cranberries support cardiovascular health by preventing plaque formation on the arterial walls. Vitamin E and heart-healthy monounsaturated fats are both abundant in almonds.*

CHERRY VANILLA PROTEIN SMOOTHIE

Calories: 160 kCal | Protein: 10 g | Carbohydrates: 25 g | Sugar: 18 g | Fat: 2 g | Fiber: 3 g | Cholesterol: 0 mg | Sodium: 75 mg | Phosphorus: 60 mg | Potassium: 320 mg.

8 min | 0 min | 2

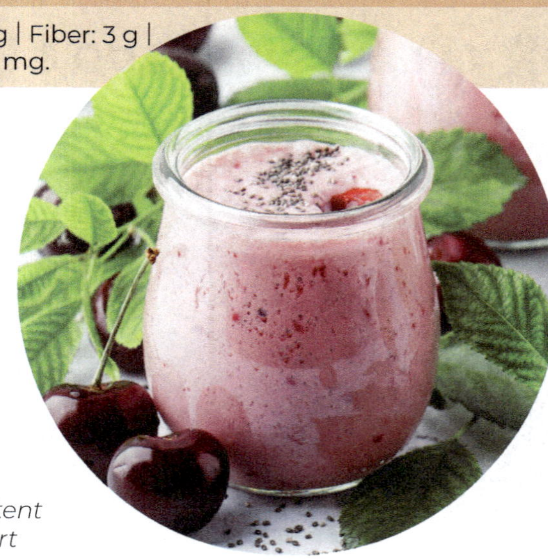

Ingredients:

- 1 cup fresh cherries, pitted
- One teaspoon of vanilla extract
- One scoop of plant-based protein powder (e.g., pea protein)
- 1 cup almond milk

Directions:

1. Combine cherries, vanilla extract, protein powder, and almond milk in a blender.
2. Blend until creamy and smooth.
3. Pour into glasses and serve immediately.

Heart-Healthy Benefits: *Anthocyanins, abundant in cherries and linked to less inflammation and a lower risk of heart disease, are potent antioxidants. Plant-based protein is associated with a healthier heart profile than animal proteins.*

BLACKBERRY MINT FRESHNESS JUICE

Calories: 55 kCal | Protein: 1 g | Carbohydrates: 13 g | Sugar: 7 g | Fat: 0,5 g | Fiber: 5 g | Cholesterol: 0 mg | Sodium: 5 mg | Phosphorus: 20 mg | Potassium: 170 mg.

10 min | 0 min | 2

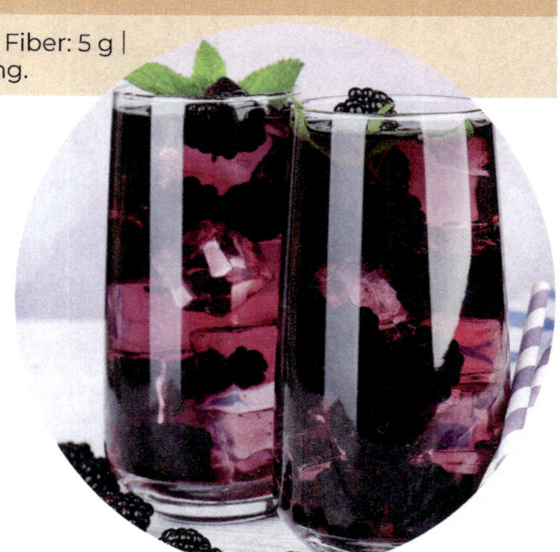

Ingredients:

- 1 cup fresh blackberries
- 8-10 mint leaves
- 1 cup cold water

Directions:

1. In a blender, combine blackberries, mint leaves, and water.
2. Blend until smooth.
3. To remove the seeds, strain the juice, then serve it cold.

Heart-Healthy Benefits: *Blackberries have high anthocyanin content, an antioxidant beneficial for heart health. Mint promotes healthy cholesterol levels.*

Heart-Healthy Grains & Morning Proteins

TOFU & SPINACH BREAKFAST BURRITO

Calories: 220 kCal | Protein: 9 g | Carbohydrates: 33 g | Sugar: 2 g | Fat: 7 g | Fiber: 5 g | Cholesterol: 0 mg | Sodium: 200 mg | Phosphorus: 150 mg | Potassium: 300 mg.

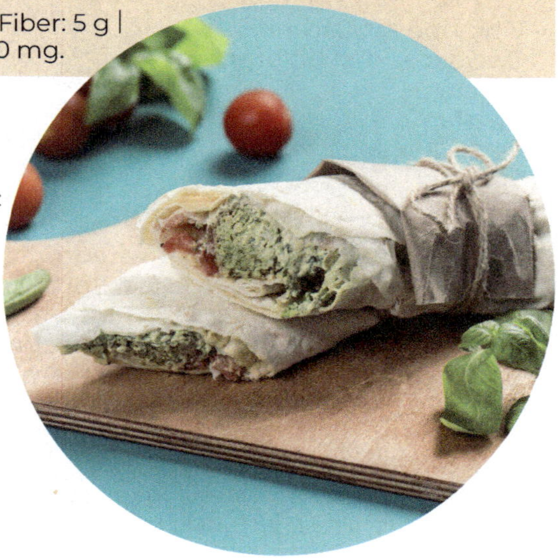

15 min | 10 min | 4

Ingredients:

- 1 cup firm tofu, crumbled
- 2 cups fresh spinach, chopped
- Four whole-grain tortillas
- One tablespoon of olive oil
- 1/4 teaspoon turmeric
- 1/4 teaspoon black pepper

Directions:

1. The olive oil should be heated in a skillet over medium heat. Turmeric and tofu crumbles should be added. Cook until tofu is lightly golden.
2. Add chopped spinach and cook until wilted.
3. Add black pepper, then turn off the heat.
4. Spoon the tofu and spinach mixture onto the center of each tortilla. Roll up to form a burrito.

Heart-Healthy Benefits: *Excellent plant-based protein sources that can lower cholesterol include tofu. Spinach is high in potassium and magnesium, which benefit heart health.*

RASPBERRY CHIA OVERNIGHT OATS

Calories: 190 kCal | Protein: 6 g | Carbohydrates: 32 g | Sugar: 6 g | Fat: 5 g | Fiber: 9 g | Cholesterol: 0 mg | Sodium: 80 mg | Phosphorus: 90 mg | Potassium: 150 mg.

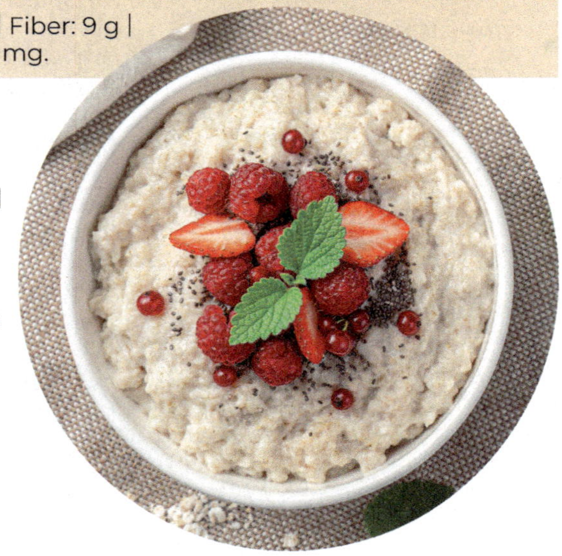

10 min | 0 min (refrigerate overnight) | 4

Ingredients:

- 2 cups almond milk
- 1 cup rolled oats
- Two tablespoons chia seeds
- 1 cup fresh raspberries
- One tablespoon of maple syrup
- 1/2 teaspoon vanilla extract

Directions:

1. Combine the almond milk, rolled oats, chia seeds, maple syrup, and vanilla extract in a bowl.
2. Gently fold in the raspberries.
3. Divide the mixture into four jars or containers. Seal and refrigerate overnight.
4. In the morning, stir the oats and enjoy the cold.

Heart-Healthy Benefits: *Omega-3 fatty acids are abundant in chia seeds and are suitable for heart health. Soluble fiber, which is present in oats, may lower harmful cholesterol.*

AVOCADO & POACHED EGG TOAST

Calories: 230 kCal | Protein: 9 g | Carbohydrates: 25 g | Sugar: 2 g | Fat: 11 g | Fiber: 7 g | Cholesterol: 186 mg | Sodium: 150 mg | Phosphorus: 60 mg | Potassium: 450 mg.

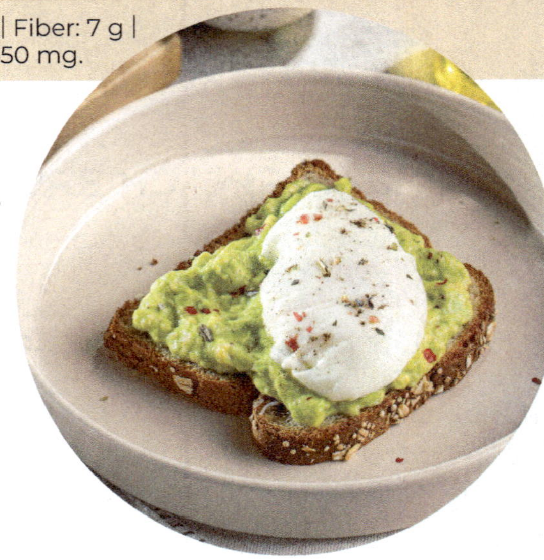

10 min | 5 min | 2

INGREDIENTS:

- One ripe avocado
- Two slices of whole-grain bread
- Two large eggs
- One tablespoon of white vinegar
- A sprinkle of black sesame seeds
- Fresh parsley, chopped, for garnish

DIRECTIONS:

1. Mash the avocado and set aside.
2. Toast the bread slices until they're golden brown.
3. Add a pot of water to a simmer and white vinegar to poach the eggs. Create a whirlpool using a spoon, and gently drop an egg into the center—Poach for about 3 minutes or until the desired doneness. Repeat with the other egg.
4. Spread the mashed avocado on each toast slice. Top with a poached egg, sprinkle with black sesame seeds and garnish with parsley.

Heart-Healthy Benefits: *Avocado contains monounsaturated fats, which are known for their heart-healthy benefits. Whole grains, such as bread, can help improve blood cholesterol levels.*

CINNAMON APPLE BARLEY PORRIDGE

Calories: 180 kCal | Protein: 4 g | Carbohydrates: 42 g | Sugar: 10 g | Fat: 1 g | Fiber: 8 g | Cholesterol: 0 mg | Sodium: 5 mg | Phosphorus: 55 mg | Potassium: 135 mg.

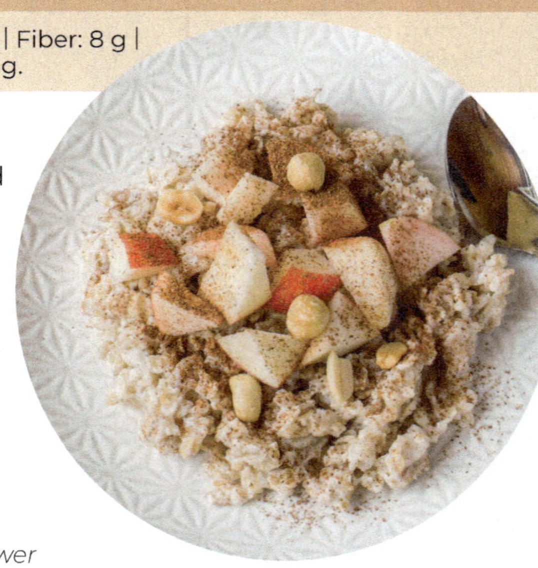

10 min | 40 min | 4

INGREDIENTS:

- 1 cup pearl barley
- 2 cups water
- Two medium apples, diced
- One teaspoon of ground cinnamon
- One tablespoon of maple syrup
- 1/4 cup almond milk

DIRECTIONS:

1. Rinse barley under cold water and drain.
2. Bring the water to a boil in a pot. Add barley, reduce heat, cover, and simmer for 30 minutes.
3. Add diced apples and cinnamon to the barley. Continue to cook for 10 minutes or until the apples are soft and the barley is cooked.
4. Stir in maple syrup and almond milk for added creaminess. Serve warm.

Heart-Healthy Benefits: *A nutritious grain called barley can help lower cholesterol and lower the chance of developing heart disease. Apples are an excellent source of vitamin C and dietary fiber.*

NOTES

MORNING GLORY OAT BOWL

Calories: 190 kCal | Protein: 6 g | Carbohydrates: 35 g | Sugar: 10 g | Fat: 4 g | Fiber: 6 g | Cholesterol: 0 mg | Sodium: 10 mg | Phosphorus: 75 mg | Potassium: 240 mg.

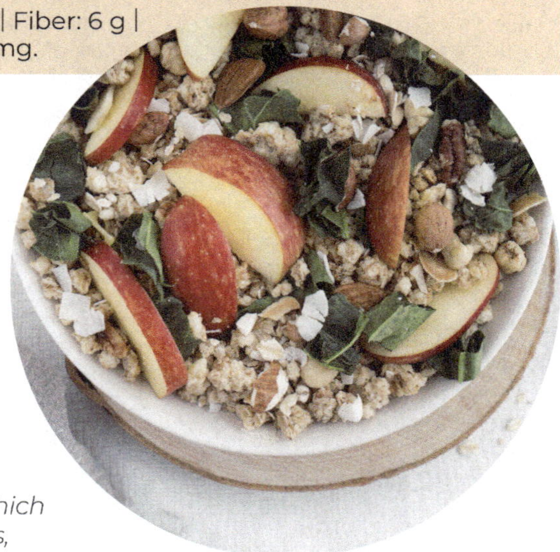

10 min | 5 min | 4

INGREDIENTS:

- 1 cup rolled oats
- 2 cups water
- One tablespoon of chia seeds
- One apple, diced
- A handful of walnuts
- A drizzle of maple syrup or honey

DIRECTIONS:

1. n a pot, bring water to a boil and add the oats. Simmer for 5 minutes or until oats are cooked.
2. Stir in chia seeds and let them thicken for 2-3 minutes.
3. Serve in bowls with diced apple, walnuts, and a drizzle of maple syrup or honey.

Heart-Healthy Benefits: *Oats are known to contain beta-glucans, which can help reduce cholesterol levels. Walnuts have omega-3 fatty acids, which are beneficial for heart health.*

NUTTY QUINOA BREAKFAST DELIGHT

Calories: 210 kCal | Protein: 8 g | Carbohydrates: 30 g | Sugar: 8 g | Fat: 6 g | Fiber: 4 g | Cholesterol: 0 mg | Sodium: 55 mg | Phosphorus: 150 mg | Potassium: 310 mg.

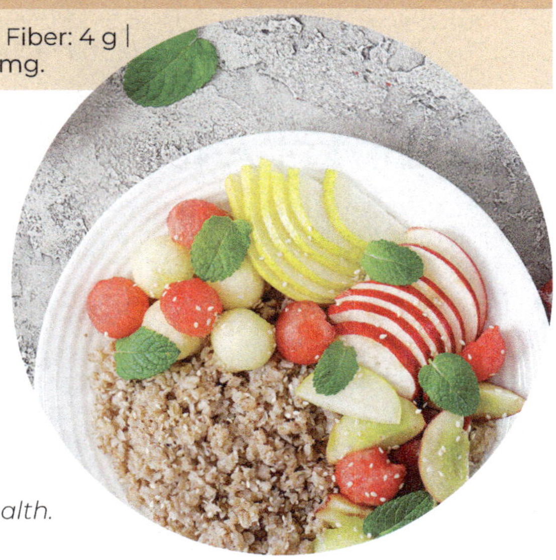

5 min | 15 min | 4

INGREDIENTS:

- 1 cup quinoa
- 2 cups almond milk
- Two tablespoons of almond butter
- A handful of sliced almonds and pistachios
- Fresh berries for topping

DIRECTIONS:

1. Rinse the quinoa under cold water.
2. Bring almond milk to a boil in a pot. Add quinoa and simmer on low heat for 15 minutes or until quinoa is cooked and fluffy.
3. Stir in almond butter.
4. Serve topped with sliced nuts and fresh berries.

Heart-Healthy Benefits: *Quinoa is a complete protein rich in magnesium, which can help relax blood vessels, promoting heart health. Almonds and pistachios are heart-healthy nuts.*

ALMOND CRUNCH YOGURT PARFAIT

Calories: 220 kCal | Protein: 8 g | Carbohydrates: 30 g | Sugar: 9 g | Fat: 8 g | Fiber: 4 g | Cholesterol: 0 mg | Sodium: 70 mg | Phosphorus: 100 mg | Potassium: 200 mg.

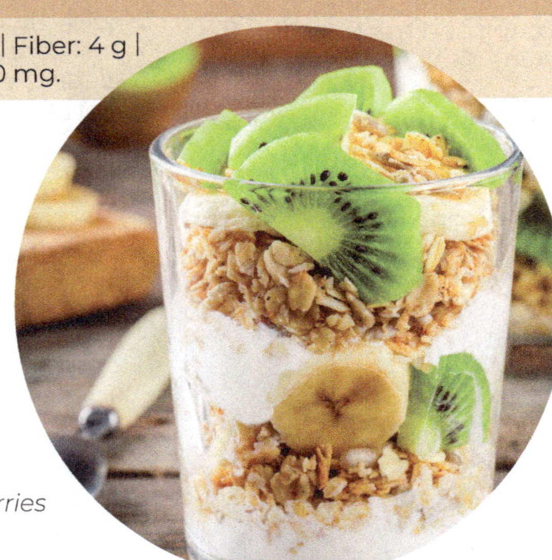

7 min | 0 min | 2

INGREDIENTS:

- 2 cups unsweetened almond yogurt
- 1/2 cup granola (ensure no added sugars)
- 1/4 cup sliced almonds
- Fresh berries for topping

DIRECTIONS:

1. In serving glasses, layer almond yogurt, granola, and almonds.
2. Repeat layers until the glass is filled.
3. Top with fresh berries.

Heart-Healthy Benefits: *Almonds are a heart-healthy source of unsaturated fats and have been shown to lower bad cholesterol. Berries are packed with antioxidants that support cardiovascular health.*

SAVORY VEGGIE BREAKFAST MUFFINS

Calories: 110 kCal | Protein: 4 g | Carbohydrates: 20 g | Sugar: 2 g | Fat: 3 g | Fiber: 4 g | Cholesterol: 0 mg | Sodium: 150 mg | Phosphorus: 120 mg | Potassium: 180 mg.

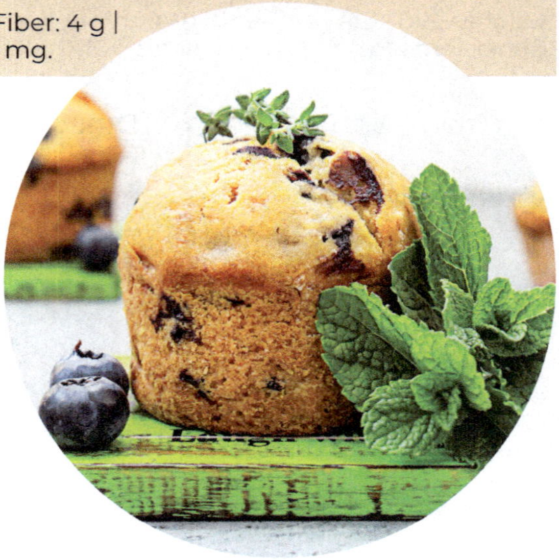

15 min | 20 min | 6

INGREDIENTS:

- 1 cup whole wheat flour
- 1/2 cup almond milk
- 1 cup mixed vegetables (like bell peppers, zucchini, and carrots), finely diced
- One teaspoon of baking powder
- 1/4 teaspoon black pepper
- 1/4 teaspoon salt
- One tablespoon of olive oil

DIRECTIONS:

1. Preheat oven to 375°F (190°C) and prepare a muffin tin with non-stick spray or liners.
2. Combine whole wheat flour, baking powder, salt, and pepper in a large bowl.
3. Olive oil and almond milk should only be blended barely.
4. Fold in the diced vegetables.
5. Equally, distribute the batter among the muffin cups.
6. Bake for 20 minutes or until a toothpick inserted into the center comes clean.

Heart-Healthy Benefits: *Whole wheat flour provides whole grains that can help regulate blood pressure and reduce the risk of heart disease. The use of olive oil instead of butter reduces saturated fats.*

MEDITERRANEAN FETA & VEGGIE OMELETTE

Calories: 210 kCal | Protein: 13 g | Carbohydrates: 5 g | Sugar: 3 g | Fat: 16 g | Fiber: 1 g | Cholesterol: 370 mg | Sodium: 300 mg | Phosphorus: 90 mg | Potassium: 230 mg.

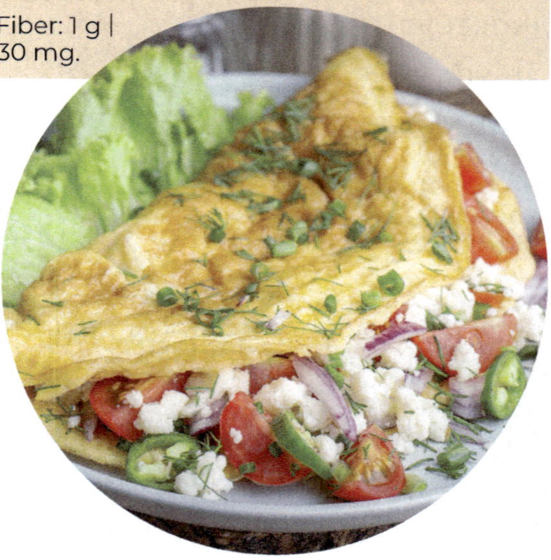

10 min | 8 min | 2

INGREDIENTS:

- Four large eggs
- 1/4 cup diced tomatoes
- 1/4 cup diced bell peppers
- 1/4 cup crumbled feta cheese (choose low-fat, low-sodium variety)
- Two tablespoons chopped fresh basil
- One tablespoon of olive oil
- Salt and pepper to taste (use salt sparingly)

DIRECTIONS:

1. The eggs should be whisked in a bowl with some salt and pepper.
2. In a non-stick skillet over medium heat, warm the olive oil.
3. Pour the eggs and let them cook without stirring for about 2 minutes.
4. Sprinkle the tomatoes, bell peppers, and feta cheese evenly over one-half of the omelet.
5. Fold the other half over the fillings and cook for 2-3 minutes.
6. Place the warm omelet on a platter and garnish with fresh basil.

Heart-Healthy Benefits: *Tomatoes are a great source of antioxidants, particularly lycopene, linked to many heart health benefits, including reduced risk of heart disease. Olive oil contains monounsaturated fats that are considered heart-healthy.*

SUNRISE BERRY BUCKWHEAT PANCAKES

Calories: 180 kCal | Protein: 5 g | Carbohydrates: 35 g | Sugar: 6 g | Fat: 3 g | Fiber: 4 g | Cholesterol: 0 mg | Sodium: 80 mg | Phosphorus: 120 mg | Potassium: 180 mg.

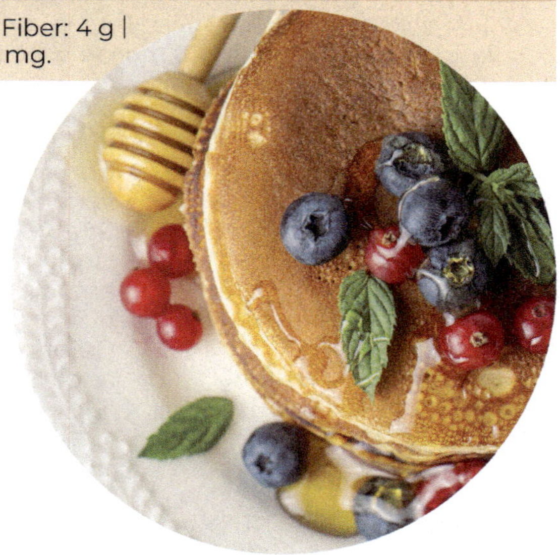

15 min | 10 min | 4

INGREDIENTS:

- 1 cup buckwheat flour
- 1 cup almond milk
- 1/2 cup mixed berries (like blueberries, raspberries, and strawberries)
- One teaspoon of baking powder
- One tablespoon of maple syrup
- One teaspoon of vanilla extract
- Coconut oil for cooking (use sparingly)

DIRECTIONS:

1. Combine buckwheat flour, baking powder, almond milk, maple syrup, and vanilla extract in a bowl. Mix until smooth.
2. Gently fold in the mixed berries.
3. Lightly coat a non-stick skillet with coconut oil and heat it over medium heat
4. For each pancake, pour 1/4 cup of batter into the grill. Cook until bubbles appear on the surface, then turn and cook until golden.
5. If desired, serve pancakes warm with extra berries or a drizzle of maple syrup.

Heart-Healthy Benefits: *Despite its name, Buckwheat is not a type of wheat but a gluten-free seed. It's rich in fiber and antioxidants, which can help improve blood flow and prevent heart disease.*

QUICK BREAKFAST IDEAS FOR BUSY MORNINGS

TROPICAL FRUIT & NUT SALAD

Calories: 180 kCal | Protein: 3 g | Carbohydrates: 30 g | Sugar: 18 g | Fat: 7 g | Fiber: 4 g | Cholesterol: 0 mg | Sodium: 10 mg | Phosphorus: 80 mg | Potassium: 400 mg.

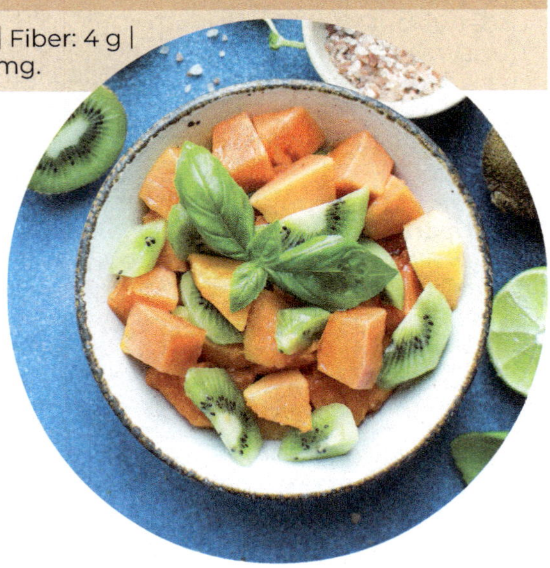

10 min | 0 min | 4

INGREDIENTS:

- 1 cup diced mango
- 1 cup diced papaya
- 1/2 cup chopped kiwi
- 1/4 cup toasted cashews
- 1/4 cup toasted coconut flakes
- Juice of 1 lime
- Fresh mint leaves for garnish

DIRECTIONS:

1. In a large bowl, combine mango, papaya, and kiwi.
2. Add lime juice, then gently toss to combine.
3. Top with toasted cashews and coconut flakes.
4. Garnish with fresh mint leaves before serving.

Heart-Healthy Benefits: *Mangoes, papayas, and kiwis are high in fiber, vitamins, and antioxidants. Cashews contain heart-healthy monounsaturated fats and have been linked to improving blood lipid levels.*

VANILLA CHIA & BERRY PUDDING POT

Calories: 160 kCal | Protein: 4 g | Carbohydrates: 20 g | Sugar: 8 g | Fat: 8 g | Fiber: 8 g | Cholesterol: 0 mg | Sodium: 60 mg | Phosphorus: 100 mg | Potassium: 150 mg.

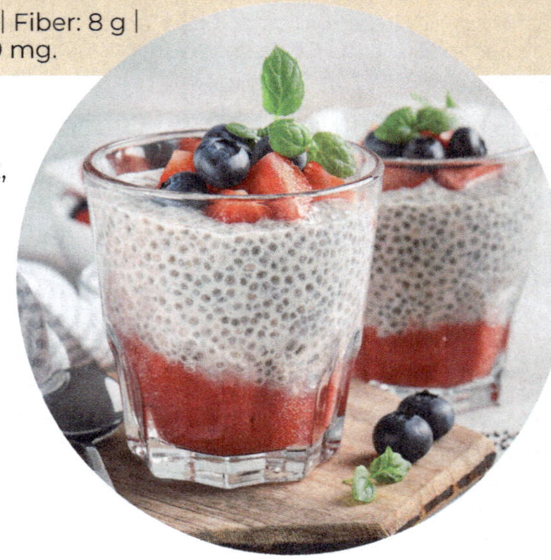

10 min (plus soaking time) | 0 min | 4

INGREDIENTS:

- 1/4 cup chia seeds
- 1 cup almond milk
- One teaspoon of vanilla extract
- Two tablespoons of maple syrup
- 1/2 cup mixed berries (raspberries, blueberries, strawberries)

DIRECTIONS:

1. Combine chia seeds, almond milk, vanilla extract, and maple syrup. Stir well.
2. Until the mixture thickens, cover and chill for at least 4 hours or overnight.
3. Before serving, stir the pudding and divide into serving pots.
4. Top with mixed berries.

Heart-Healthy Benefits: *Omega-3 fatty acids, abundant in chia seeds, can lower the risk of heart disease. Berries are packed with antioxidants linked to lower cholesterol levels and blood pressure.*

BREEZY BANANA & PEANUT BUTTER ROLL-UPS

Calories: 220 kCal | Protein: 6 g | Carbohydrates: 35 g | Sugar: 8 g | Fat: 7 g | Fiber: 5 g | Cholesterol: 0 mg | Sodium: 150 mg | Phosphorus: 100 mg | Potassium: 300 mg.

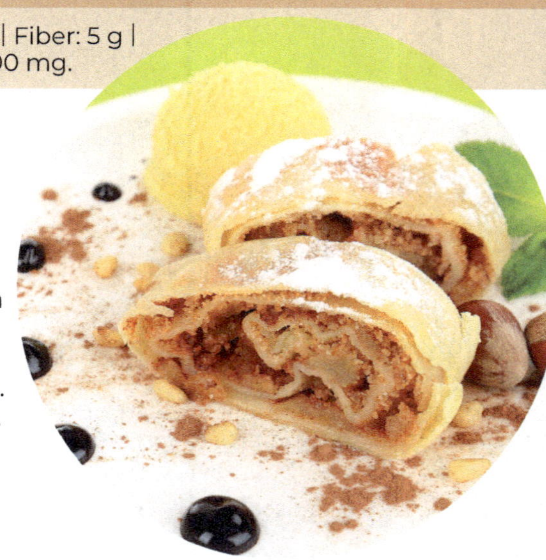

10 min | 0 min | 4

INGREDIENTS:

- Four whole-grain tortillas
- Two bananas, peeled and sliced
- Four tablespoons peanut butter (unsweetened)
- One tablespoon honey (optional)
- A sprinkle of cinnamon (optional)

DIRECTIONS:

1. Lay out the tortillas on a flat surface.
2. Spread each tortilla with a tablespoon of peanut butter.
3. Place banana slices in a line down the center of each tortilla.
4. If desired, sprinkling cinnamon and drizzling honey will be added.
5. Roll the tortilla around the fillings, slice it in half, and serve.

Heart-Healthy Benefits: *Bananas are a fantastic source of potassium, which helps control blood pressure. When consumed in moderation, peanut butter's protein and healthy fats suit the Heart.*

NOTES

MORNING MUESLI WITH DRIED FRUITS

Calories: 210 kCal | Protein: 5 g | Carbohydrates: 40 g | Sugar: 15 g | Fat: 4 g | Fiber: 5 g | Cholesterol: 0 mg | Sodium: 60 mg | Phosphorus: 100 mg | Potassium: 250 mg.

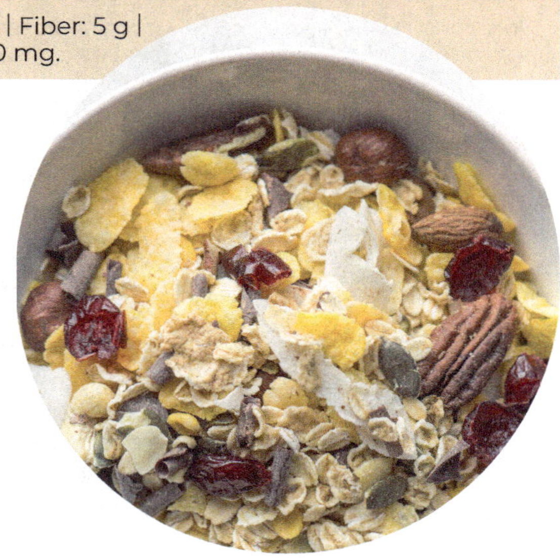

10 min (plus soaking time) | 0 min | 4

INGREDIENTS:

- 1 cup muesli
- 1 1/2 cups almond milk
- 1/4 cup mixed dried fruits (raisins, apricots, dates), chopped
- One tablespoon honey
- 1/4 teaspoon ground cinnamon

DIRECTIONS:

1. Combine muesli, almond milk, dried fruits, love, and cinnamon in a bowl.
2. Mix well, cover, and refrigerate overnight.
3. Before serving, stir it well and add more almond milk if desired.
4. Serve chilled.

Heart-Healthy Benefits: *Muesli, a mix of oats and other grains, is fiber-rich and supports heart health. Dried fruits provide essential vitamins and minerals. However, be mindful of portion sizes due to their sugar content. As always, it's essential to consult with a healthcare professional before significantly changing your diet. It ensures that your dietary choices are suitable for your specific health needs.*

SESAME & DATE MORNING ENERGY BALLS

Calories: 120 kCal | Protein: 3 g | Carbohydrates: 18 g | Sugar: 14 g | Fat: 5 g | Fiber: 3 g | Cholesterol: 0 mg | Sodium: 20 mg | Phosphorus: 50 mg | Potassium: 200 mg.

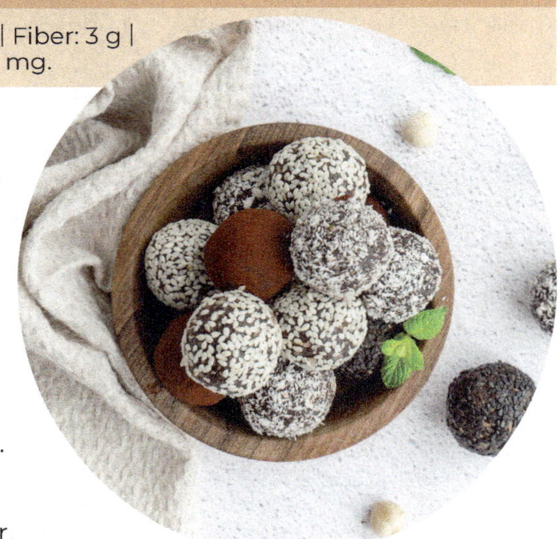

15 min | 0 min | 6 (2 balls per serving)

INGREDIENTS:

- 1 cup dates, pitted
- 1/2 cup almonds
- One tablespoon of sesame seeds
- 1/2 teaspoon vanilla extract
- A pinch of salt
- Two tablespoons water

DIRECTIONS:

1. Combine dates, almonds, sesame seeds, vanilla extract, and salt in a food processor.
2. Pulse until the mixture becomes crumbly.
3. Slowly add water while the machine runs until the mixture starts coming together.
4. Roll the mixture into bite-sized balls after transferring it to a bowl.
5. Before serving, place the balls on a dish covered with parchment paper and chill for at least an hour.

Heart-Healthy Benefits: *Dates are a natural sweetener that provides essential nutrients and fiber. Almonds and sesame seeds contribute heart-healthy fats and antioxidants that support cardiovascular health. Consult a healthcare or nutritional professional to ensure these recipes meet individual dietary needs.*

NOTES

WARM CINNAMON APPLE & RYE TOAST

Calories: 180 kCal | Protein: 5 g | Carbohydrates: 35 g | Sugar: 10 g | Fat: 4 g | Fiber: 5 g | Cholesterol: 0 mg | Sodium: 120 mg | Phosphorus: 60 mg | Potassium: 130 mg.

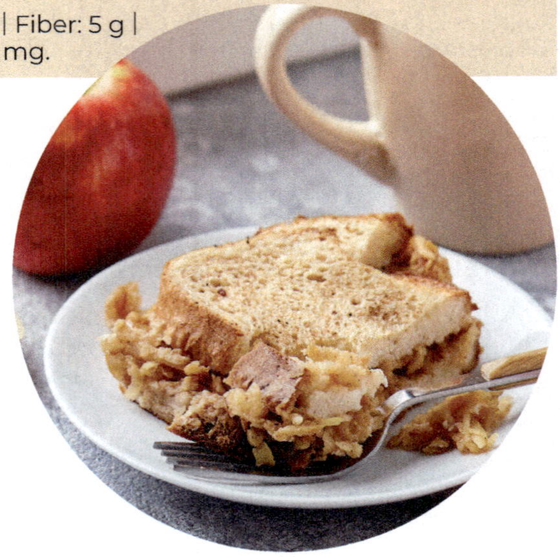

10 min | 10 min | 4

INGREDIENTS:

- Four slices of whole-grain rye bread
- Two medium apples, thinly sliced
- One tablespoon honey
- 1/2 teaspoon ground cinnamon
- One tablespoon of olive oil
- Fresh mint leaves for garnish (optional)

DIRECTIONS:

1. In a skillet, heat olive oil over medium heat.
2. Add the apple slices, honey, and cinnamon. Cook, stirring occasionally, until the apples are tender and slightly caramelized, about 5-7 minutes.
3. While the apples are cooking, toast the rye bread slices.
4. Top each toast with the warm cinnamon apple mixture.
5. If preferred, garnish with fresh mint leaves before serving.

Heart-Healthy Benefits: *Rye bread made from whole grains helps lower blood sugar levels and lower the risk of heart disease. Apples are a great source of dietary fiber and antioxidants for your Heart.*

CHERRY ALMOND MORNING MUFFINS

Calories: 180 kCal | Protein: 5 g | Carbohydrates: 35 g | Sugar: 10 g | Fat: 3 g | Fiber: 4 g | Cholesterol: 0 mg | Sodium: 80 mg | Phosphorus: 70 mg | Potassium: 110 mg.

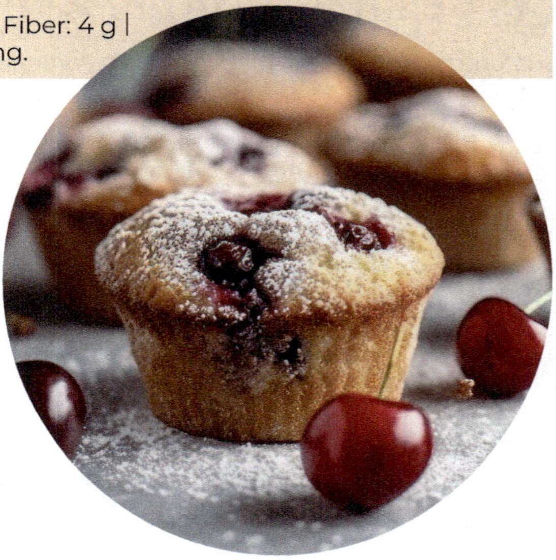

15 min | 20 min | 6

INGREDIENTS:

- 1 cup whole wheat flour
- 1/2 cup rolled oats
- 1/2 teaspoon baking soda
- 1/4 cup honey
- 1/2 cup unsweetened almond milk
- 1/2 cup fresh cherries, pitted and chopped
- 1/4 cup almonds, chopped
- One teaspoon of vanilla extract

DIRECTIONS:

1. Preheat oven to 375°F (190°C) and line a muffin tin with paper liners.
2. Mix whole wheat flour, rolled oats, and baking soda in a bowl.
3. In another bowl, combine honey, almond milk, and vanilla extract.
4. Stir constantly, and gradually add the wet liquid to the dry ingredients.
5. Gently fold in cherries and almonds.
6. Make sure to fill the muffin pans with the batter equally.
7. A toothpick put into a muffin should come out clean after 20 minutes in the oven.
8. Allow to cool before serving.

Heart-Healthy Benefits: *Cherries contain antioxidants called anthocyanins, which can reduce inflammation and lower cholesterol. Almonds add healthy fats and vitamin E, both beneficial for heart health.*

HEARTY SALADS

AVOCADO & QUINOA POWER SALAD

Calories: 230 kCal | Protein: 6 g | Carbohydrates: 30 g | Sugar: 3 g | Fat: 12 g | Fiber: 7 g | Cholesterol: 0 mg | Sodium: 150 mg | Phosphorus: 100 mg | Potassium: 400 mg.

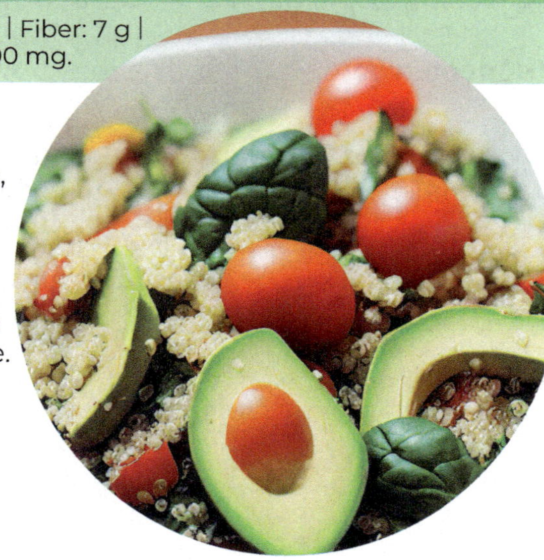

10 min | 10 min | 4

INGREDIENTS:

- 1 cup cooked quinoa (follow package instructions)
- One ripe avocado, diced
- 1 cup cherry tomatoes, halved
- 1/2 cup cucumber, diced
- 1/4 cup red onion, finely chopped
- Two tablespoons of olive oil
- Juice of 1 lime
- Salt and pepper to taste

DIRECTIONS:

1. Combine cooked quinoa, avocado, cherry tomatoes, cucumber, and red onion in a large bowl.
2. Combine the olive oil, lime juice, salt, and pepper in another bowl.
3. The dressing will cover the quinoa mixture; gently toss to incorporate.
4. Offer cold.

Heart-Healthy Benefits: *Avocado is loaded with monounsaturated fats and potassium, which support heart health. Quinoa is a complete protein and a good source of magnesium and fiber, essential for cardiovascular health.*

GRILLED ZUCCHINI & PINE NUT MEDLEY

Calories: 140 kCal | Protein: 3 g | Carbohydrates: 8 g | Sugar: 2 g | Fat: 12 g | Fiber: 2 g | Cholesterol: 0 mg | Sodium: 20 mg | Phosphorus: 60 mg | Potassium: 250 mg.

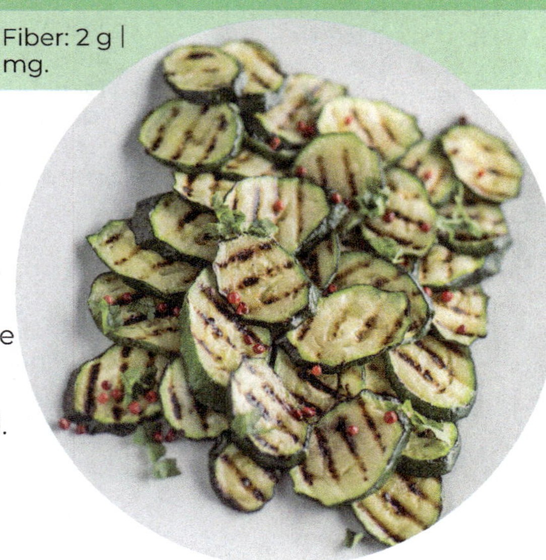

10 min | 8 min | 4

INGREDIENTS:

- Two medium zucchinis, sliced lengthwise
- 1/4 cup pine nuts, toasted
- Two tablespoons of olive oil
- One tablespoon of lemon juice
- 1/4 teaspoon black pepper
- Fresh basil leaves for garnish

DIRECTIONS:

1. Preheat a grill or grill pan over medium heat.
2. Brush zucchini slices with one tablespoon of olive oil and grill for about 4 minutes on each side.
3. Transfer to a serving plate. Sprinkle with pine nuts.
4. Combine the remaining olive oil, lemon juice, and pepper in a bowl. Drizzle over zucchini and pine nuts.
5. Garnish with fresh basil leaves before serving.

Heart-Healthy Benefits: *Zucchini is a low-calorie vegetable with dietary fiber and antioxidants. Pine nuts contain monounsaturated fats that can help lower harmful cholesterol levels.*

WARM MUSHROOM & LENTIL SALAD

Calories: 210 kCal | Protein: 10 g | Carbohydrates: 25 g | Sugar: 4 g | Fat: 8 g | Fiber: 8 g | Cholesterol: 0 mg | Sodium: 70 mg | Phosphorus: 180 mg | Potassium: 400 mg.

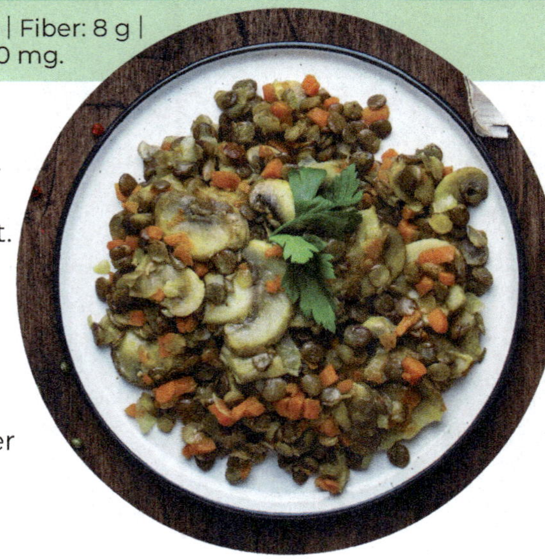

10 min | 25 min | 4

INGREDIENTS:

- 1 cup cooked lentils
- 2 cups sliced mushrooms (e.g., cremini or white button)
- Two tablespoons of olive oil
- One garlic clove, minced
- Two tablespoons of balsamic vinegar
- Salt and pepper to taste
- Fresh parsley for garnish

DIRECTIONS:

1. In a large skillet, heat olive oil over medium heat.
2. Add garlic and sauté until fragrant.
3. Add mushrooms and cook until tender.
4. Stir in the cooked lentils and balsamic vinegar, and cook for 3 minutes.
5. Season with salt and pepper.
6. Add fresh parsley as a garnish after transferring to serving bowls.

Heart-Healthy Benefits: *Lentils are a rich source of protein and fiber, which can help reduce cholesterol levels. Mushrooms are known for their anti-inflammatory properties.*

BERRY BURST SPINACH SALAD

Calories: 180 kCal | Protein: 4 g | Carbohydrates: 15 g | Sugar: 8 g | Fat: 12 g | Fiber: 4 g | Cholesterol: 0 mg | Sodium: 60 mg | Phosphorus: 80 mg | Potassium: 300 mg.

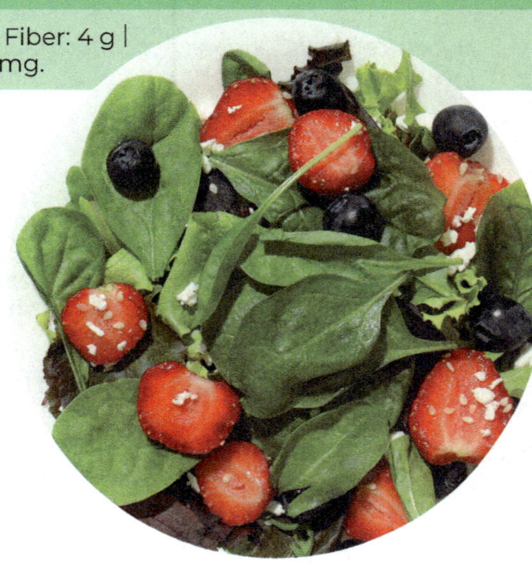

10 min | 0 min | 4

INGREDIENTS:

- 4 cups baby spinach
- 1 cup mixed berries (strawberries, blueberries, raspberries)
- 1/4 cup chopped walnuts
- Two tablespoons of olive oil
- One tablespoon of lemon juice
- One teaspoon honey
- Salt and pepper to taste

DIRECTIONS:

1. Combine spinach, mixed berries, and chopped walnuts in a large bowl.
2. Whisk together olive oil, lemon juice, honey, salt, and pepper in a small bowl.
3. Add the dressing to the salad and gently stir.
4. Serve immediately.

Heart-Healthy Benefits: *Berries are packed with antioxidants that benefit heart health. Spinach contains magnesium and folate, which play a role in maintaining a healthy cardiovascular system.*

NOTES

Wraps, Sandwiches & More: Low-Sodium Variations

GOLDEN TURMERIC CHICKEN PITA POCKETS

Calories: 280 kCal | Protein: 20 g | Carbohydrates: 30 g | Sugar: 3 g | Fat: 9 g | Fiber: 4 g | Cholesterol: 40 mg (for chicken option) | Sodium: 150 mg | Phosphorus: 200 mg | Potassium: 400 mg.

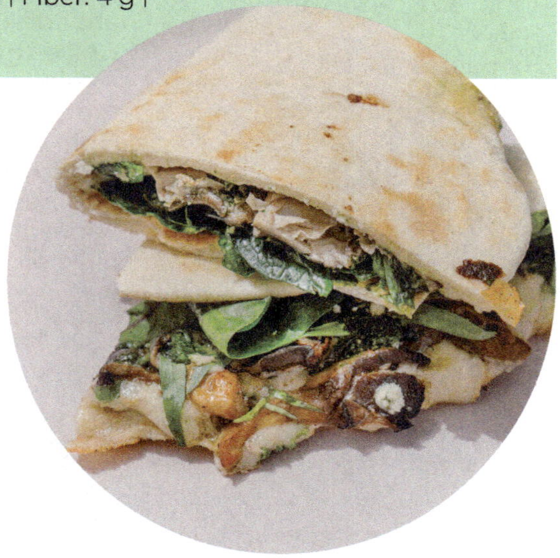

15 min | 15 min | 4

Ingredients:

- Two chicken breasts, diced (or tofu/chickpea alternative)
- Two teaspoons of turmeric powder
- Two tablespoons of olive oil
- Four pita pockets
- 1 cup fresh spinach
- 1/4 cup Greek yogurt (or plant-based yogurt)

Directions:

1. In a bowl, toss chicken/tofu/chickpeas with turmeric powder.
2. Heat olive oil over medium heat in a skillet and cook the chicken/tofu/chickpeas until fully cooked.
3. Cut the top of the pita pockets and fill each with an equal amount of the chicken/tofu/chickpea mix.
4. Add fresh spinach and a dollop of yogurt.

Heart-Healthy Benefits: *Turmeric contains curcumin, known for its anti-inflammatory effects, which can benefit heart health. Spinach is rich in folate and other vitamins and minerals that support cardiovascular health.*

COOL CUCUMBER & TUNA SALAD SANDWICH

Calories: 220 kCal | Protein: 18 g | Carbohydrates: 30 g | Sugar: 4 g | Fat: 4 g | Fiber: 5 g | Cholesterol: 30 mg | Sodium: 150 mg | Phosphorus: 180 mg | Potassium: 320 mg.

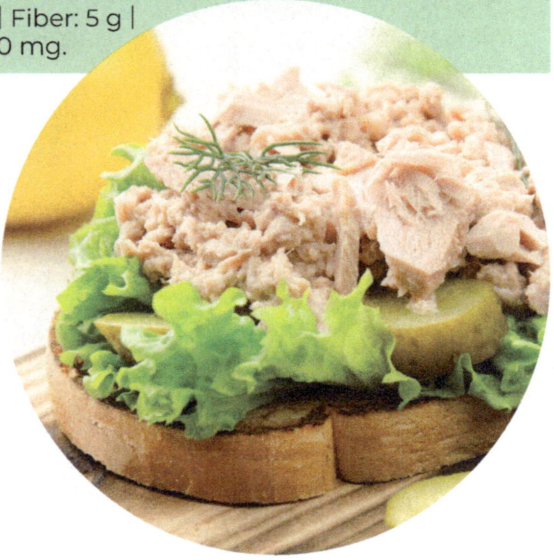

10 min | 0 min | 4

Ingredients:

- One can (15 oz) of tuna in water, drained
- One medium cucumber, finely diced
- Two tablespoons vegan mayonnaise
- One tablespoon of Dijon mustard
- Two tablespoons fresh dill, chopped
- Eight slices whole grain bread
- Fresh lettuce

Directions:

1. Mix the drained tuna, diced cucumber, vegan mayonnaise, Dijon mustard, and dill in a bowl.
2. Season with salt and pepper to taste.
3. Spread the tuna mix onto four slices of bread.
4. Add fresh lettuce and top with the remaining bread slices.

Heart-Healthy Benefits: *Tuna is an excellent source of omega-3 fatty acids that benefit heart health. Whole grain bread provides dietary fiber, which helps in cholesterol management.*

GRILLED EGGPLANT & TOMATO CIABATTA

Calories: 250 kCal | Protein: 8 g | Carbohydrates: 40 g | Sugar: 6 g | Fat: 7 g | Fiber: 8 g | Cholesterol: 0 mg | Sodium: 180 mg | Phosphorus: 150 mg | Potassium: 480 mg.

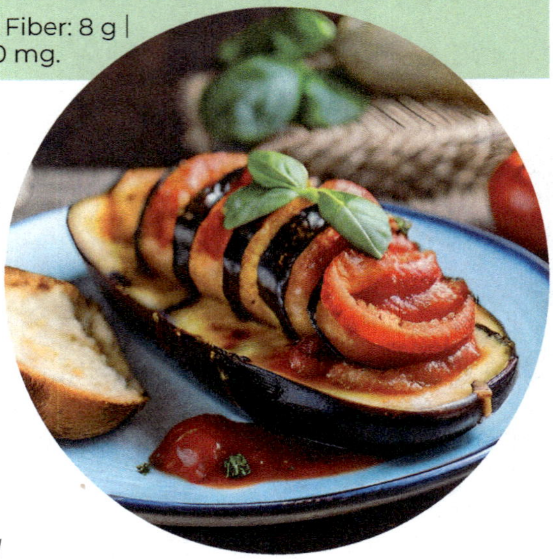

15 min | 10 min | 4

INGREDIENTS:

- One large eggplant, sliced
- Two large tomatoes, sliced
- Four ciabatta rolls
- Two tablespoons of olive oil
- Fresh basil leaves
- Salt and pepper to taste

DIRECTIONS:

1. Preheat a grill or grill pan.
2. Slices of eggplant are brushed with olive oil, and salt and pepper are added.
3. Grill eggplant slices for about 4 minutes on each side or until tender.
4. Open ciabatta rolls and layer with grilled eggplant, tomato slices, and fresh basil.
5. Serve after adding a little more olive oil, if preferred.

Heart-Healthy Benefits: *Eggplants are rich in fiber, antioxidants, and potassium, which can benefit heart health. The antioxidant lycopene, associated with a lower risk of heart disease, is abundant in tomatoes.*

OPEN-FACED AVOCADO & RADISH TOASTIE

Calories: 180 kCal | Protein: 4 g | Carbohydrates: 15 g | Sugar: 8 g | Fat: 12 g | Fiber: 4 g | Cholesterol: 0 mg | Sodium: 60 mg | Phosphorus: 80 mg | Potassium: 300 mg.

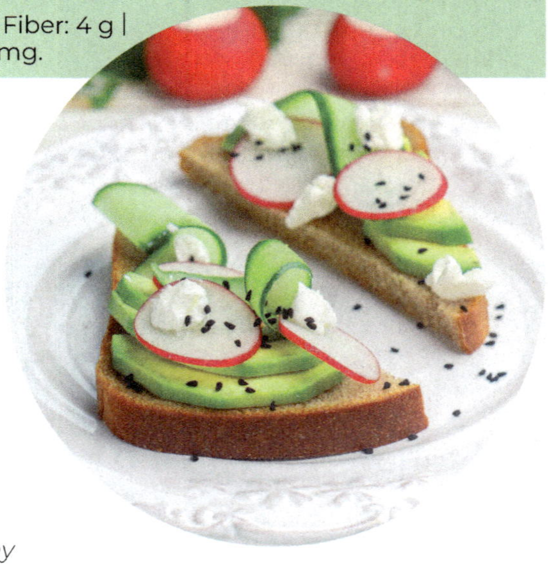

10 min | 2 min (toasting) | 4

INGREDIENTS:

- Four slices of whole-grain bread
- Two ripe avocados
- 6-8 radishes, thinly sliced
- One tablespoon of lemon juice
- Fresh chives, chopped for garnish
- Salt and pepper to taste

DIRECTIONS:

1. Toast the whole grain bread slices.
2. In a bowl, mash the avocados and combine with the lemon juice. Add salt and pepper to taste.
3. On the toasted pieces, equally, distribute the mashed avocado.
4. Top with radish slices and garnish with chopped chives.

Heart-Healthy Benefits: *Avocados are a good source of heart-healthy monounsaturated fats. Whole grains provide essential nutrients and dietary fiber, which benefit cardiovascular health.*

NOTES

BALSAMIC MUSHROOM & ARUGULA BAGUETTE

Calories: 220 kCal | Protein: 7 g | Carbohydrates: 40 g | Sugar: 4 g | Fat: 4 g | Fiber: 6 g | Cholesterol: 0 mg | Sodium: 200 mg | Phosphorus: 90 mg | Potassium: 350 mg.

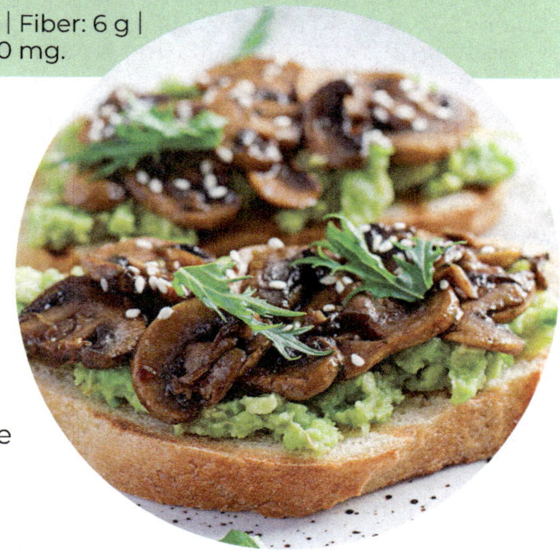

10 min | 15 min | 4

INGREDIENTS:

- 2 cups sliced mushrooms (e.g., button or cremini)
- One tablespoon of olive oil
- Two tablespoons of balsamic vinegar
- One garlic clove, minced
- 1 cup arugula
- One whole grain baguette, sliced into four portions
- Salt and pepper to taste

DIRECTIONS:

1. Heat the olive oil in a pan and sauté the garlic until fragrant.
2. Add the sliced mushrooms and cook until browned.
3. Pour balsamic vinegar and stir, letting the mushrooms soak up the flavor.
4. Season with salt and pepper.
5. Lay out the baguette slices, place arugula on each, then top with the balsamic mushrooms.

Heart-Healthy Benefits: *Mushrooms are low in calories and provide essential nutrients, including selenium, potassium, riboflavin, niacin, and vitamin D. Arugula, with its peppery flavor, is rich in nitrate beneficial for heart health.*

QUICK PREP + PACKABLE OPTIONS

HERB ROASTED VEGGIE & COUSCOUS COMBO

Calories: 260 kCal | Protein: 8 g | Carbohydrates: 50 g | Sugar: 2 g | Fat: 4 g | Fiber: 5 g | Cholesterol: 0 mg | Sodium: 150 mg | Phosphorus: 110 mg | Potassium: 330 mg.

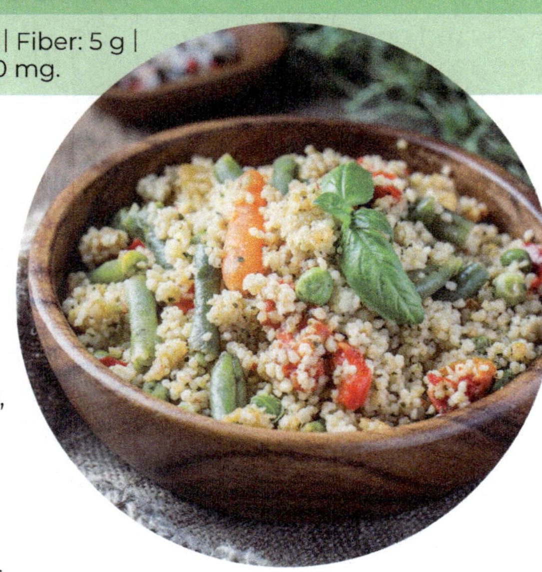

10 min | 20 min | 4

INGREDIENTS:

- 1 cup couscous
- 2 cups mixed vegetables (e.g., zucchini, bell peppers, cherry tomatoes)
- One tablespoon of olive oil
- One teaspoon mixed dried herbs (like rosemary, thyme, basil)
- Salt and pepper to taste
- 2 cups vegetable broth or water

DIRECTIONS:

1. Preheat oven to 400°F (200°C). Toss mixed vegetables with olive oil, dried herbs, salt, and pepper.
2. Spread the vegetables on a baking sheet and roast for 15-20 minutes or until tender and slightly golden.
3. While the vegetables are roasting, bring vegetable broth or water to a boil and add the couscous. Cover and let sit off the heat for 5 minutes.
4. Fluff the couscous with a fork and mix in the roasted vegetables.

Heart-Healthy Benefits: *Couscous is a good source of fiber and protein. Roasted vegetables offer a range of vitamins and antioxidants beneficial for heart health.*

TOMATO BASIL MOZZARELLA STICKS

Calories: 120 kCal | Protein: 2 g | Carbohydrates: 8 g | Sugar: 5 g | Fat: 9 g | Fiber: 2 g | Cholesterol: 0 mg | Sodium: 120 mg | Phosphorus: 30 mg | Potassium: 290 mg.

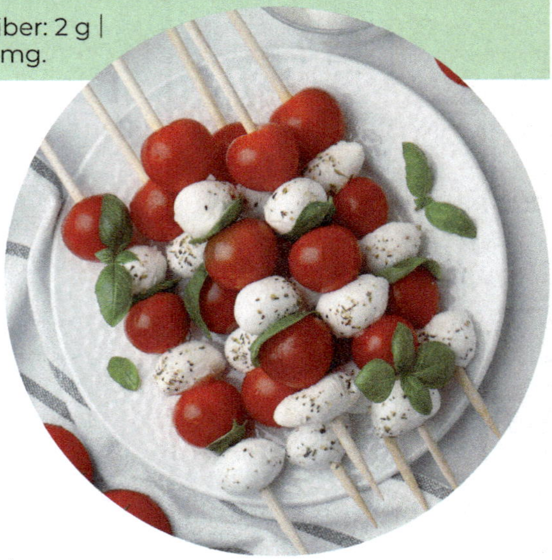

10 min | 0 min | 4

INGREDIENTS:

- Two large tomatoes, sliced into rounds
- 1/2 cup fresh basil leaves
- Vegan mozzarella cheese cut into rounds
- One tablespoon of olive oil
- One tablespoon of balsamic vinegar
- Salt and pepper to taste

DIRECTIONS:

1. Arrange the tomato slices on a serving platter.
2. Top each tomato slice with a basil leaf and vegan mozzarella.
3. Drizzle with olive oil and balsamic vinegar.
4. Season with salt and pepper and serve.

Heart-Healthy Benefits: *Tomatoes are rich in lycopene, an antioxidant known to promote heart health. Olive oil is a source of monounsaturated fats, which can help lower harmful cholesterol levels.*

CHICKPEA & CUCUMBER SALAD BOWL

Calories: 210 kCal | Protein: 8 g | Carbohydrates: 27 g | Sugar: 5 g | Fat: 8 g | Fiber: 7 g | Cholesterol: 0 mg | Sodium: 150 mg | Phosphorus: 120 mg | Potassium: 450 mg.

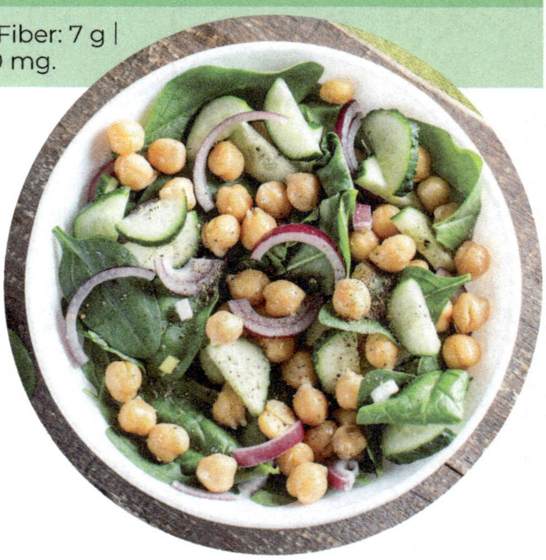

15 min | 0 min | 4

INGREDIENTS:

- 2 cups chickpeas, cooked and drained
- One large cucumber, diced
- One red bell pepper, diced
- 1/4 cup fresh parsley, chopped
- Two tablespoons of olive oil
- One tablespoon of lemon juice
- Salt and pepper to taste

DIRECTIONS:

1. Combine chickpeas, cucumber, red bell pepper, and parsley in a large bowl.
2. Whisk together olive oil, lemon juice, salt, and pepper in a separate smaller bowl.
3. Pour the dressing over the salad and mix well.

Heart-Healthy Benefits: *Chickpeas provide plant-based protein and soluble fiber, which can help lower cholesterol. Cucumbers are a good source of vitamin K and antioxidants.*

NOTES

HONEY DRIZZLED STRAWBERRY & ALMOND PLATE

Calories: 90 kCal | Protein: 2 g | Carbohydrates: 14 g | Sugar: 10 g | Fat: 4 g | Fiber: 3 g | Cholesterol: 0 mg | Sodium: 0 mg | Phosphorus: 40 mg | Potassium: 220 mg.

5 min | 0 min | 4

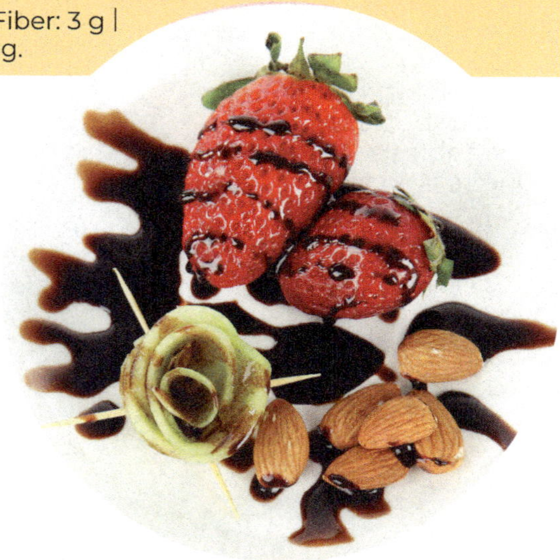

INGREDIENTS:

- 2 cups strawberries, halved
- ¼ cup almonds, toasted and roughly chopped
- Two tablespoons honey

DIRECTIONS:

1. Arrange strawberry halves on a plate.
2. Sprinkle toasted almonds over strawberries.
3. Drizzle with honey just before serving. Add fresh spinach and a dollop of yogurt.

Heart-Healthy Benefits: *Strawberries are rich in antioxidants, particularly vitamin C and manganese, which support heart health. Almonds are an excellent source of monounsaturated fats, known to lower harmful cholesterol levels.*

ROASTED BELL PEPPER STRIPS WITH HUMMUS

Calories: 190 kCal | Protein: 5 g | Carbohydrates: 20 g | Sugar: 4 g | Fat: 10 g | Fiber: 6 g | Cholesterol: 0 mg | Sodium: 130 mg | Phosphorus: 70 mg | Potassium: 290 mg.

10 min | 20 min | 4

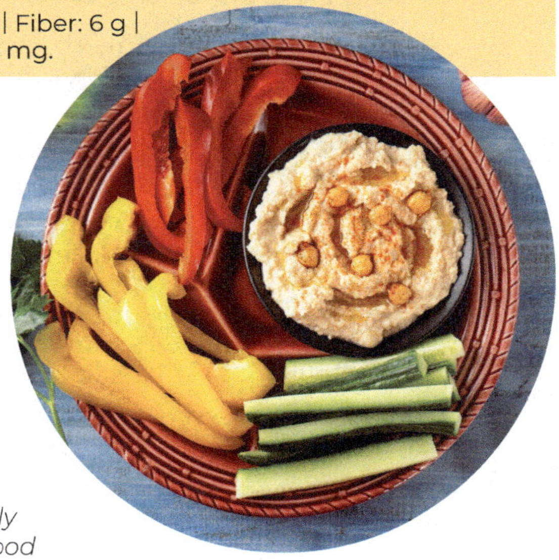

INGREDIENTS:

- Three bell peppers (red, yellow, and green) sliced into strips
- One tablespoon of olive oil
- 1 cup hummus (store-bought or homemade)
- Fresh parsley for garnish

DIRECTIONS:

1. Preheat oven to 400°F (205°C).
2. Toss bell pepper strips in olive oil and spread on a baking sheet.
3. Roast for 20 minutes or until edges are slightly charred.
4. Serve roasted bell pepper strips with hummus and garnish with fresh parsley.

Heart-Healthy Benefits: *Bell peppers are rich in vitamins, particularly Vitamin C, and antioxidants. Hummus, made from chickpeas, is a good source of protein and dietary fiber, which can aid in lowering cholesterol.*

NOTES

TANGY APPLE SLICES WITH PEANUT SPREAD

Calories: 180 kCal | Protein: 4 g | Carbohydrates: 25 g | Sugar: 18 g | Fat: 8 g | Fiber: 4 g | Cholesterol: 0 mg | Sodium: 5 mg | Phosphorus: 50 mg | Potassium: 210 mg.

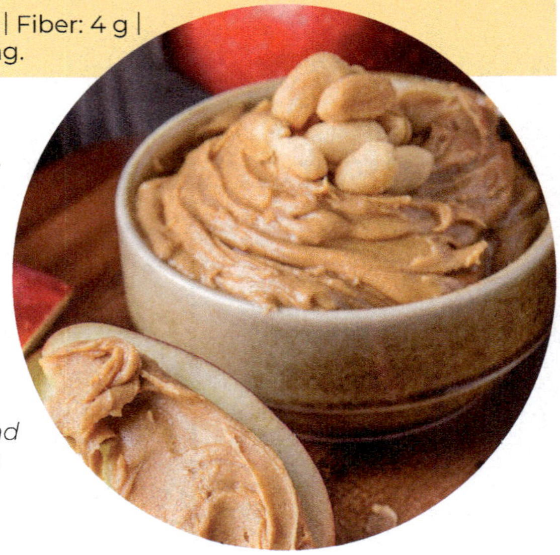

5 min | 0 min | 4

INGREDIENTS:

- Two large apples, cored and sliced
- Four tablespoons peanut butter (unsalted)
- One tablespoon honey
- One teaspoon cinnamon

DIRECTIONS:

1. In a small bowl, mix peanut butter with honey and cinnamon.
2. Spread the mixture onto apple slices before serving.

Heart-Healthy Benefits: *Apples are a great source of dietary fiber and vitamin C. Peanut butter provides protein and potassium, which can help lower the risk of high blood pressure.*

LEAN PROTEINS + VEGETABLE PAIRINGS

MUSHROOM & QUINOA STUFFED BELL PEPPERS

Calories: 180 kCal | Protein: 6 g | Carbohydrates: 30 g | Sugar: 5 g | Fat: 6 g | Fiber: 6 g | Cholesterol: 0 mg | Sodium: 80 mg | Phosphorus: 240 mg | Potassium: 460 mg.

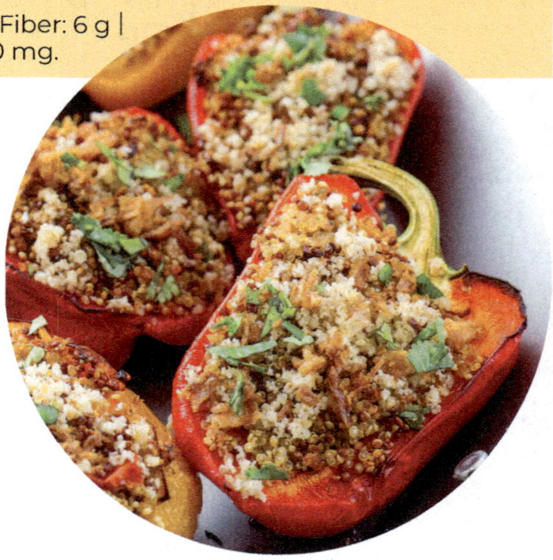

20 min | 30 min | 4

INGREDIENTS:

- Four large bell peppers, tops removed and seeded
- 1 cup cooked quinoa
- 1 cup mushrooms, finely chopped
- One small onion, finely chopped
- Two cloves garlic, minced
- Two tablespoons of olive oil
- One teaspoon dried oregano
- Salt to taste (mind the sodium)
- Freshly ground black pepper

DIRECTIONS:

1. Preheat oven to 375°F (190°C).
2. Warm up the olive oil in a skillet over medium heat. Add onions and garlic, sautéing until translucent.
3. Add mushrooms, oregano, salt, and pepper. Cook until mushrooms are tender.
4. Mix in cooked quinoa, combining well.
5. Fill each bell pepper with the quinoa-mushroom mixture.
6. Place stuffed peppers in a baking dish and cover with aluminum foil.
7. Bake for 30 minutes or until peppers are tender.
8. Serve immediately.

Heart-Healthy Benefits: *Quinoa has all nine essential amino acids and is a complete protein. It's also high in fiber, which is beneficial for heart health. Mushrooms provide crucial vitamins and minerals, and bell peppers are rich in antioxidants and Vitamin C, which can help maintain a healthy heart.*

BROCCOLI & CAULIFLOWER IN LEMON VINAIGRETTE

Calories: 100 kCal | Protein: 3 g | Carbohydrates: 10 g | Sugar: 3 g | Fat: 7 g | Fiber: 4 g | Cholesterol: 0 | Sodium: 40 mg | Phosphorus: 60 mg | Potassium: 300 mg.

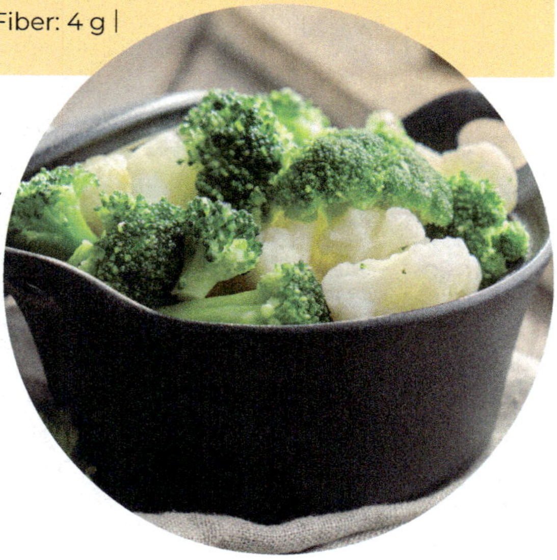

10 min | 7 min | 4

INGREDIENTS:

- 2 cups broccoli florets
- 2 cups cauliflower florets
- Zest and juice of 1 lemon
- Two tablespoons of olive oil
- Salt to taste (mind the sodium)
- Freshly ground black pepper
- One tablespoon of chopped fresh parsley

DIRECTIONS:

1. Bring a pot of water to boil. Add broccoli cauliflower, and blanch for 2-3 minutes or until slightly tender but crunchy. Drain and place in a large bowl.
2. Whisk together lemon zest, lemon juice, olive oil, salt, and pepper in a small bowl.
3. Pour the lemon vinaigrette over the blanched vegetables and toss to coat.
4. Garnish with fresh parsley before serving.

Heart-Healthy Benefits: *Broccoli and cauliflower are cruciferous vegetables known for their cancer-fighting properties and ability to reduce inflammation, which is beneficial for heart health. Lemon contains antioxidants and can help improve the elasticity of blood vessels.*

THESE DISHES ARE NOT JUST DELIGHTFUL IN TASTE BUT ARE ALSO DESIGNED TO NOURISH YOUR HEART AND OVERALL HEALTH. REMEMBER, USING FRESH INGREDIENTS, MAINTAINING BALANCED PORTIONS, AND ENJOYING A DIVERSE DIET FOR THE BEST HEART HEALTH OUTCOMES ARE ESSENTIAL.

HEART-HEALTHY PASTAS + GRAINS

WHOLE WHEAT SPAGHETTI WITH BASIL PESTO

Calories: 350 kCal | Protein: 12 g | Carbohydrates: 49 g | Sugar: 3 g | Fat: 12 g | Fiber: 6 g | Cholesterol: 5 mg | Sodium: 250 mg | Phosphorus: 180 mg | Potassium: 290 mg.

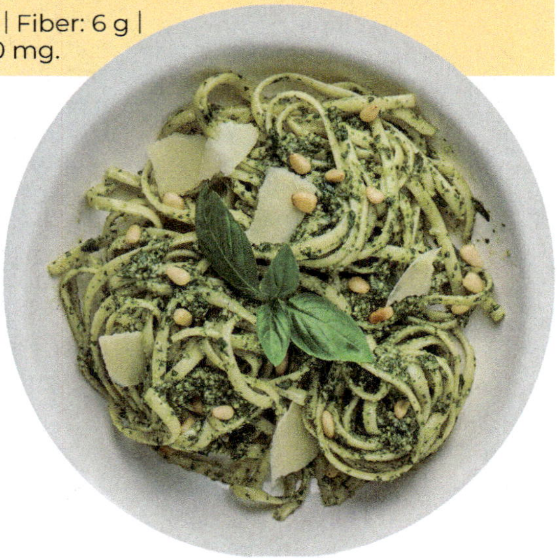

10 min | 15 min | 4

INGREDIENTS:

- Eight oz. whole wheat spaghetti
- 2 cups fresh basil leaves
- Two cloves garlic
- Two tablespoons pine nuts (or walnuts)
- 1/4 cup grated Parmesan cheese (optional for vegans)
- Two tablespoons extra virgin olive oil
- 1/4 cup water
- Salt, to taste (remember to monitor sodium levels)
- One tablespoon of lemon juice

DIRECTIONS:

1. Boil a large pot of water and cook the spaghetti according to package instructions.
2. While the pasta cooks, combine the basil, garlic, nuts, and cheese in a blender or food processor.
3. Slowly drizzle in the olive oil and water as the machine runs until a smooth consistency is reached.
4. Season with salt (sparingly) and lemon juice.
5. Drain and add the cooked pasta back to the saucepan.
6. Mix in the basil pesto until the pasta is well coated. Serve immediately.

Heart-Healthy Benefits: *Whole wheat provides dietary fiber, which is beneficial for heart health by reducing harmful cholesterol levels. A good source of monounsaturated fats believed to lower the risk of heart disease is olive oil, known to decrease heart disease risks. Basil and garlic provide antioxidants that support heart health.*

QUINOA WITH FRESH HERBS & LEMON ZEST

Calories: 200 kCal | Protein: 8 g | Carbohydrates: 35 g | Sugar: 2 g | Fat: 5 g | Fiber: 4 g | Cholesterol: 0 mg | Sodium: 70 mg | Phosphorus: 180 mg | Potassium: 320 mg.

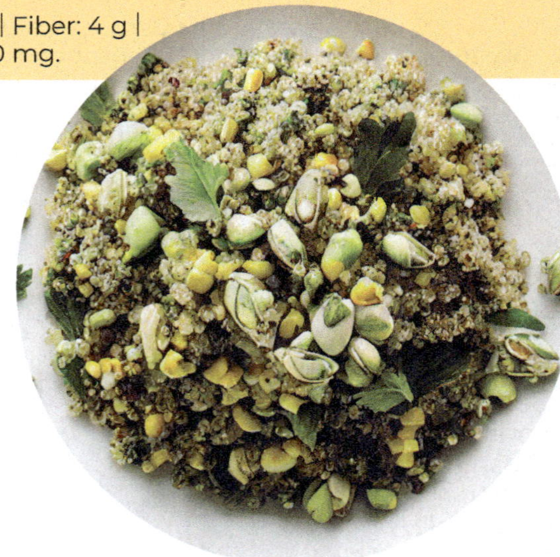

10 min | 20 min | 4

INGREDIENTS:

- 1 cup quinoa, rinsed and drained
- 2 cups water
- Zest of 1 lemon
- 1/4 cup mixed fresh herbs (parsley, cilantro, dill), finely chopped
- 1 tbsp olive oil
- Salt to taste (keep sodium below 20% per serving)

DIRECTIONS:

1. Mix the quinoa, water, and a little salt in a saucepan. Up to a boil.
2. Once quinoa is tender and water has been absorbed, reduce heat to low, cover, and simmer for 15 minutes.
3. Remove from heat, cover, and allow to stand for five minutes.
4. With a fork, fluff the quinoa, then add the lemon zest, fresh herbs, and olive oil.

Heart-Healthy Benefits: *Quinoa is a complete protein and whole grain beneficial for heart health. Fresh herbs provide antioxidants, while lemon zest adds flavor without extra sodium.*

BARLEY RISOTTO WITH ASPARAGUS TIPS

Calories: 280 kCal | Protein: 8 g | Carbohydrates: 55 g | Sugar: 3 g | Fat: 5 g | Fiber: 8 g | Cholesterol: 5 mg | Sodium: 180 mg | Phosphorus: 150 mg | Potassium: 300 mg.

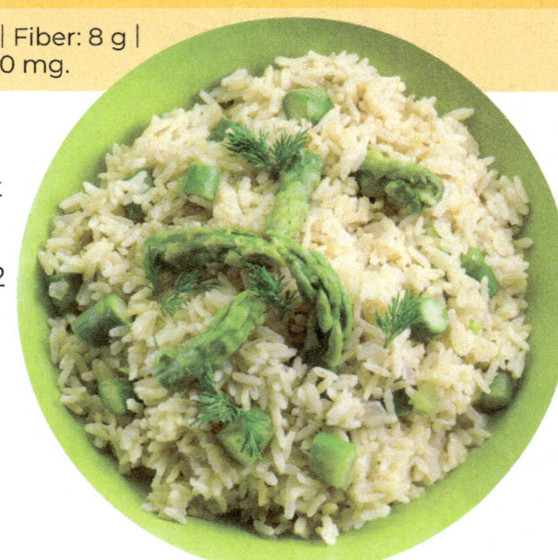

10 min | 45 min | 4

INGREDIENTS:

- 1 cup hulled barley
- 3 cups vegetable broth (low-sodium)
- 1 cup asparagus tips
- One small onion, finely chopped
- Two cloves garlic, minced
- 1 tbsp olive oil
- Salt to taste (keep sodium below 20% per serving)
- 1/4 cup grated Parmesan cheese (optional)
- Freshly ground black pepper

DIRECTIONS:

1. Olive oil should be heated in a pot over medium heat. Sauté onions until translucent, then add garlic.
2. Add barley to the pot and stir for 2 minutes. Gradually add vegetable broth one cup at a time, allowing each cup to absorb before adding the next.
3. Halfway through, add asparagus tips. Continue to cook until barley is tender and creamy.
4. On top, season with salt and freshly ground black pepper. Garnish with Parmesan cheese if desired.

Heart-Healthy Benefits: *Barley has been linked to lower cholesterol levels, which benefits heart health. Asparagus provides essential nutrients and antioxidants.*

NOTES

LENTIL & VEGETABLE COUSCOUS

Calories: 270 kCal | Protein: 11 g | Carbohydrates: 48 g | Sugar: 3 g | Fat: 4 g | Fiber: 8 g | Cholesterol: 0 | Sodium: 170 mg | Phosphorus: 220 mg | Potassium: 300 mg.

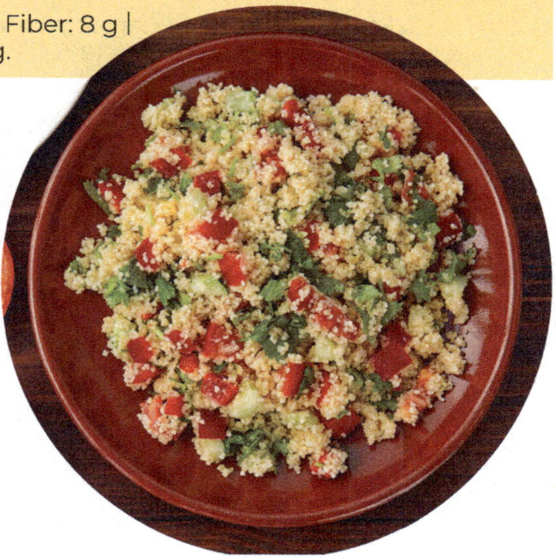

15 min | 25 min | 6

INGREDIENTS:

- 2 cups vegetable broth (low-sodium)
- 1 cup couscous
- 1 cup lentils, rinsed and drained
- One red bell pepper, diced
- One zucchini, diced
- 1/4 cup fresh parsley, chopped
- 2 tbsp olive oil
- Two cloves garlic, minced
- Juice of 1 lemon
- Salt to taste (keeping sodium below 20% per serving)

DIRECTIONS:

1. Bring 1 cup of vegetable broth to a boil in a saucepan. Add the lentils, lower the heat, and simmer for about 20 minutes or until soft.
2. Bring the remaining broth to a boil in a separate pot. Place the couscous in, turn off the heat, cover, and let stand for five minutes.
3. Olive oil is heated in a skillet at a medium temperature. Garlic, bell pepper, and zucchini should be sautéed until soft.
4. Mix cooked lentils and sautéed veggies in a big bowl, and fluff the couscous with a fork. Toss with fresh parsley and lemon juice.

Heart-Healthy Benefits: *Lentils are an excellent source of fiber and protein, beneficial for heart health. The combination of vegetables adds vitamins and antioxidants, promoting overall cardiovascular wellness.*

FLAVORFUL, LOW-FAT SAUCES & SEASONINGS

HERB-INFUSED OLIVE OIL DIP

Calories: 350 kCal | Protein: 12 g | Carbohydrates: 49 g | Sugar: 3 g | Fat: 12 g | Fiber: 6 g | Cholesterol: 5 mg | Sodium: 250 mg | Phosphorus: 180 mg | Potassium: 290 mg.

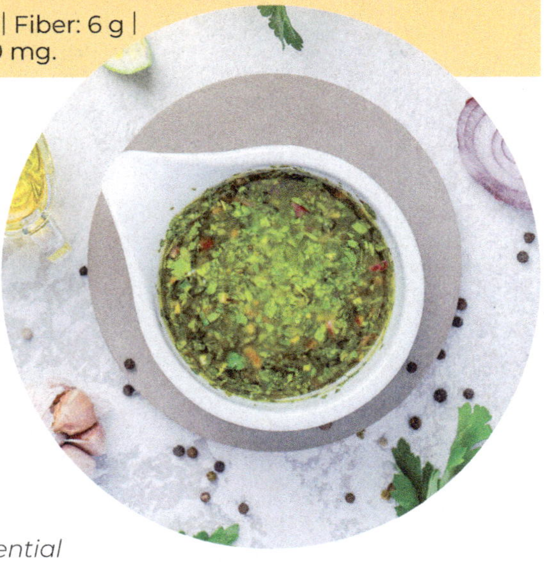

5 min | 0 min | 6

INGREDIENTS:

- 1 cup extra virgin olive oil
- Two garlic cloves, thinly sliced
- One tablespoon of fresh rosemary chopped
- One tablespoon of fresh thyme, chopped
- A pinch of black pepper
- Salt, to taste (be cautious with sodium)

DIRECTIONS:

1. Combine olive oil, garlic slices, rosemary, and thyme in a glass jar or bowl.
2. Add a little salt and black pepper for seasoning.
3. Before serving, let the mixture sit for a couple of hours to enable the flavors to mingle.
4. Stir before serving as a dip for whole grain bread or drizzled over salads.

Heart-Healthy Benefits: *as emphasized before, Olive oil provides essential monounsaturated fats for heart health. The herbs, such as rosemary and thyme, have anti-inflammatory properties and antioxidants that promote cardiovascular wellness.*
Note: Remember that the key to a heart-healthy diet is not just the individual ingredients but the overall balance and variety of foods consumed. In order to keep a healthy heart, regular exercise, stress reduction, and other lifestyle choices are essential.

ROSEMARY & LEMON VINAIGRETTE

Calories: 120 kCal | Protein: 0 g | Carbohydrates: 2 g | Sugar: 1 g | Fat: 14 g | Fiber: 0 g | Cholesterol: 0 mg | Sodium: 20 mg | Phosphorus: 5 mg | Potassium: 30 mg.

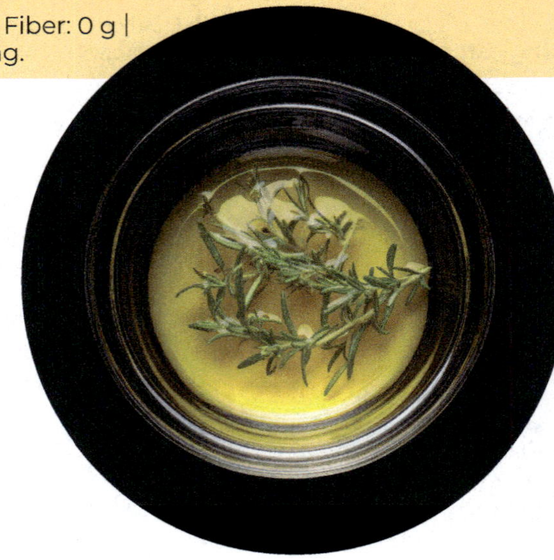

10 min | 0 min | 4

INGREDIENTS:

- 1/4 cup extra virgin olive oil
- Three tablespoons fresh lemon juice
- One teaspoon of lemon zest
- One tablespoon of fresh rosemary, finely chopped
- One garlic clove, minced
- A pinch of black pepper
- Salt, to taste (use sparingly)

DIRECTIONS:

1. Lemon juice, zest, rosemary, and garlic are combined in a basin.
2. To emulsify the dressing, olive oil should be added gradually while constantly whisking in.
3. Add a little salt and black pepper for seasoning. For up to a week, keep in the refrigerator in an airtight container.

Heart-Healthy Benefits: *Lemon provides a burst of antioxidants and vitamin C, both beneficial for heart health. The combination of olive oil and rosemary offers anti-inflammatory benefits and monounsaturated fats that support heart health.*

Note: When incorporating these recipes into your diet, remember the importance of portion control and the overall balance of your daily food intake. To improve your overall heart health, eat these heart-healthy foods in moderation, along with a balanced diet and frequent exercise.

CREAMY AVOCADO & LIME SAUCE

Calories: 80 kCal | Protein: 1 g | Carbohydrates: 5 g | Sugar: 1 g | Fat: 7 g | Fiber: 3 g | Cholesterol: 0 mg | Sodium: 20 mg | Phosphorus: 30 mg | Potassium: 250 mg.

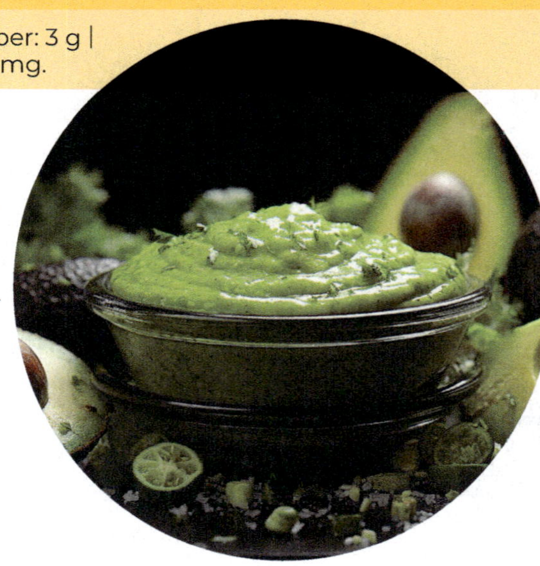

10 min | 0 min | 4

INGREDIENTS:

- One ripe avocado, pitted and peeled
- Two tablespoons of fresh lime juice
- One garlic clove, minced
- Two tablespoons fresh cilantro, chopped
- 1/4 cup water (adjust for desired consistency)
- Salt, to taste (use sparingly)
- A pinch of black pepper

DIRECTIONS:

1. Combine the avocado, lime juice, garlic, and cilantro in a blender or food processor.
2. Blend until smooth, adding water until you achieve a creamy, sauce-like consistency.
3. Season with a light touch of salt and black pepper. Serve immediately or keep in the fridge for up to a day in an airtight container.

Heart-Healthy Benefits: *Monounsaturated fats, abundant in avocados, may help lower dangerous cholesterol levels and the risk of heart disease. Lime provides vitamin C, essential for maintaining blood vessel health. Cilantro offers antioxidant properties, which can protect against heart disease.*

INCORPORATING THESE RECIPES INTO A HEART-HEALTHY LIFESTYLE IS BENEFICIAL. HOWEVER, IT'S CRUCIAL TO MAINTAIN A DIVERSE DIET RICH IN WHOLE FOODS, ENSURING YOU RECEIVE A COMPREHENSIVE RANGE OF NUTRIENTS. REGULAR EXERCISE, STRESS MANAGEMENT, REGULAR CHECK-UPS, AND MONITORING SODIUM INTAKE, ESPECIALLY FOR THOSE WITH HYPERTENSION OR HEART CONDITIONS, ARE INTEGRAL FOR HEART HEALTH.

Soup Recipes

GOLDEN LENTIL & SPINACH SOUP

Calories: 250 kCal | Protein: 14 g | Carbohydrates: 40 g | Sugar: 5 g | Fat: 3,5 g | Fiber: 15 g | Cholesterol: 0 mg | Sodium: 200 mg | Phosphorus: 200 mg | Potassium: 700 mg.

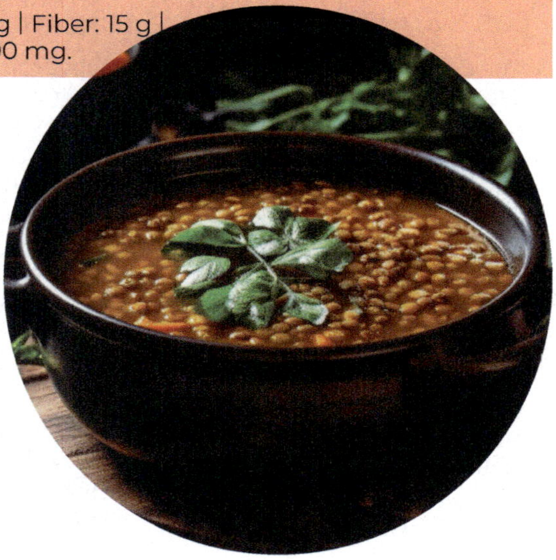

15 min | 45 min | 4

Ingredients:

- 1 tbsp olive oil
- One onion, chopped
- Two cloves garlic, minced
- One carrot, chopped
- 1 tsp turmeric
- 1 cup dried lentils, rinsed and drained
- 5 cups vegetable broth (low-sodium)
- 2 cups fresh spinach, roughly chopped
- Salt (limited) and black pepper to taste
- Lemon zest and juice from half a lemon

Directions:

1. In a large pot, olive oil is warmed over medium heat. Add onion, garlic, and carrot. Sauté for about 5 minutes until the vegetables are soft.
2. Stir in turmeric and lentils. When the mixture is at a boil, add the vegetable broth.
3. Lower the heat and let simmer for 30-35 minutes or until lentils are tender.
4. Stir in spinach and continue cooking for another 5 minutes.
5. Season with salt, pepper, lemon zest, and lemon juice before serving.

Heart-Healthy Benefits: *Lentils are a great source of fiber and protein, which are beneficial for heart health. Magnesium and folate, two vital minerals and vitamins in spinach, can help decrease blood pressure. Turmeric has anti-inflammatory properties.*

CARROT GINGER PUREE

Calories: 110 kCal | Protein: 2 g | Carbohydrates: 25 g | Sugar: 12 g | Fat: 3 g | Fiber: 5 g | Cholesterol: 0 mg | Sodium: 150 mg | Phosphorus: 80 mg | Potassium: 450 mg.

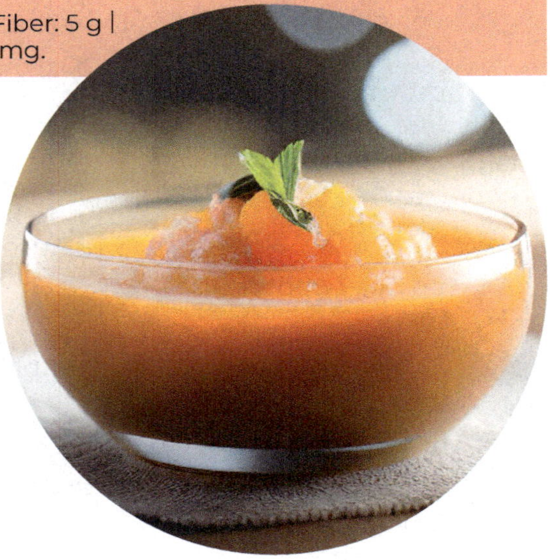

10 min | 25 min | 4

Ingredients:

- 1 tbsp olive oil
- One onion, chopped
- Two cloves garlic, minced
- Six large carrots, chopped
- 2 inches fresh ginger, peeled and minced
- 4 cups vegetable broth (low-sodium)
- Salt (limited) and black pepper to taste

Directions:

1. Olive oil is heated in a pot over a medium flame. Add onions and garlic, and sauté until translucent.
2. Add carrots, ginger, and vegetable broth. Bring to a boil.
3. Reduce the heat and let simmer for 20 minutes or until the carrots are tender.
4. Using an immersion blender, puree the soup until smooth. Alternatively, use a blender in batches.
5. Season with a pinch of salt and pepper. Serve warm.

Heart-Healthy Benefits: *Beta-carotene, abundant in carrots, may help lower the risk of heart disease. Ginger can help lower cholesterol and blood pressure. Olive oil's monounsaturated fats support a healthy heart.*

SILKY BUTTERNUT SQUASH SOUP

Calories: 160 kCal | Protein: 3 g | Carbohydrates: 30 g | Sugar: 6 g | Fat: 6 g | Fiber: 5 g | Cholesterol: 0 mg | Sodium: 160 mg | Phosphorus: 80 mg | Potassium: 550 mg.

15 min | 45 min | 4

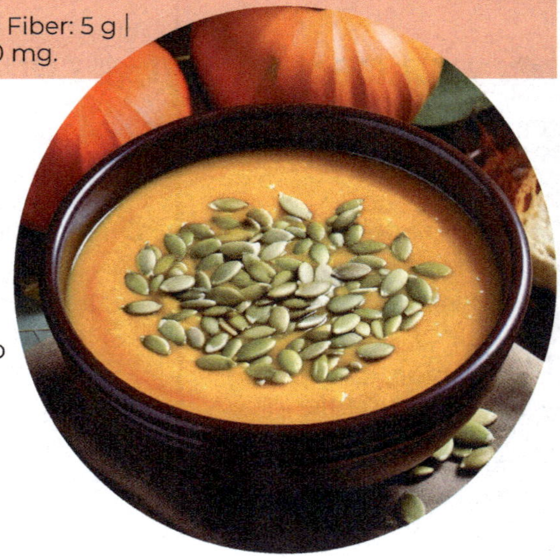

INGREDIENTS:

- 2 tbsp olive oil
- One medium butternut squash, peeled and diced
- One onion, finely chopped
- Two cloves garlic, minced
- 4 cups vegetable broth (low-sodium)
- 1/2 tsp ground nutmeg
- Salt (limited) and black pepper to taste
- 1/4 cup coconut milk (unsweetened)
- Fresh chives for garnish

DIRECTIONS:

1. Olive oil is heated in a sizable pot over a medium flame. Add onions and garlic; sauté until translucent.
2. Add butternut squash and stir for a few minutes.
3. Pour in vegetable broth, ensuring the squash is submerged. Bring to a boil.
4. Reduce heat, cover, and let simmer for 30-35 minutes or until squash is tender.
5. Puree the soup using an immersion blender until it's smooth.
6. Add coconut milk and grated nutmeg after mixing. Add a little salt and pepper for seasoning.
7. Garnish with chives before serving.

Heart-Healthy Benefits: *Butternut squash is high in fiber and potassium, which support heart health. Olive oil, rich in monounsaturated fats, improves heart health by reducing total and LDL cholesterol levels.*

SWEET CORN & BELL PEPPER CHOWDER

Calories: 200 kCal | Protein: 5 g | Carbohydrates: 40 g | Sugar: 8 g | Fat: 7 g | Fiber: 5 g | Cholesterol: 0 mg | Sodium: 140 mg | Phosphorus: 60 mg | Potassium: 500 mg.

15 min | 25 min | 4

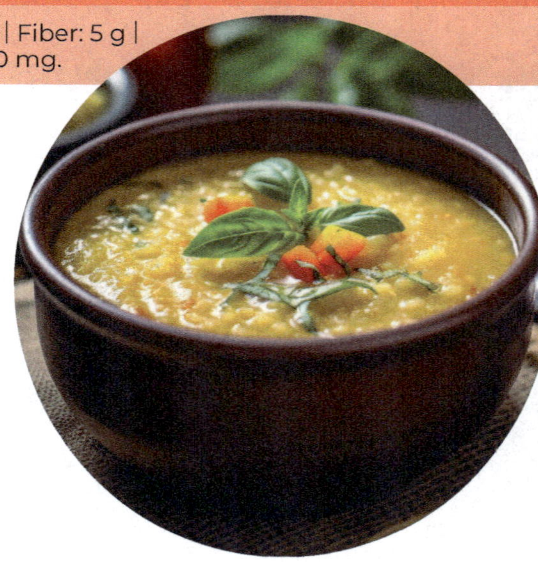

INGREDIENTS:

- 2 tbsp olive oil
- One onion, finely chopped
- Two cloves garlic, minced
- Two red bell peppers, diced
- 3 cups fresh or frozen sweet corn kernels
- 4 cups vegetable broth (low-sodium)
- 1/2 cup almond milk (unsweetened)
- Salt (limited) and black pepper to taste
- 2 tbsp fresh chives, chopped

DIRECTIONS:

1. Olive oil is heated in a sizable pot over a medium flame. Add onions, garlic, red bell peppers; sauté until vegetables soften.
2. Add corn and vegetable broth. Bring to a boil.
3. Reduce heat and let simmer for 15-20 minutes.
4. Blend until the soup after adding half of it to a blender. Combine back into the pot.
5. Stir in almond milk and season with a pinch of salt and pepper.
6. Garnish with chives before serving.

Heart-Healthy Benefits: *Beta-carotene, abundant in carrots, may help lower the risk of heart disease. Ginger can help lower cholesterol and blood pressure. Olive oil's monounsaturated fats support a healthy heart.*

COOL CUCUMBER & AVOCADO GAZPACHO

Calories: 130 kCal | Protein: 3 g | Carbohydrates: 15 g | Sugar: 5 g | Fat: 9 g | Fiber: 6 g | Cholesterol: 0 mg | Sodium: 120 mg | Phosphorus: 60 mg | Potassium: 400 mg.

20 min | 0 min | 4

Ingredients:

- Two large cucumbers, peeled and diced
- One ripe avocado, pitted and diced
- Two cloves garlic
- 1/4 cup fresh lime juice
- 2 cups vegetable broth (low-sodium)
- 1/4 cup fresh dill, chopped
- Salt (limited) and black pepper to taste

Directions:

1. Combine cucumbers, avocado, garlic, lime juice, and vegetable broth in a blender. Blend until smooth.
2. Chill the soup in the refrigerator for at least 2 hours.
3. Add the chopped dill and season with salt and pepper just before serving.

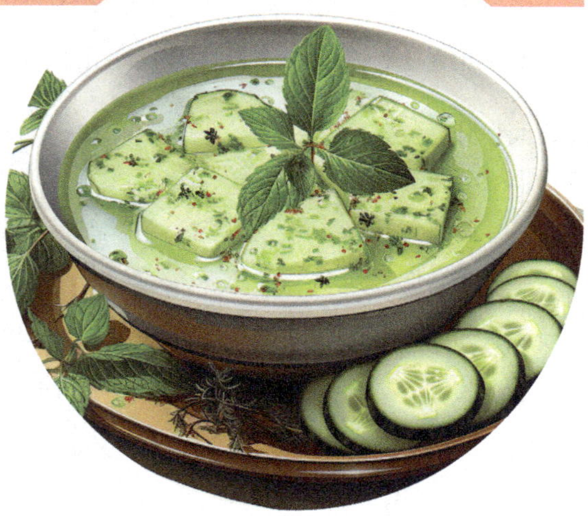

Heart-Healthy Benefits: *Avocado is a nutrient powerhouse that provides monounsaturated fatty acids and heart-healthy fats. Cucumbers contain antioxidants, including flavonoids and tannins, which prevent the accumulation of harmful free radicals, supporting heart health.*

ROASTED RED BEET AND DILL SOUP

Calories: 160 kCal | Protein: 4 g | Carbohydrates: 28 g | Sugar: 12 g | Fat: 6 g | Fiber: 5 g | Cholesterol: 0 mg | Sodium: 140 mg | Phosphorus: 70 mg | Potassium: 500 mg.

15 min | 45 min | 4

Ingredients:

- Three large red beets, peeled and diced
- 2 tbsp olive oil
- One onion, chopped
- Three cloves garlic, minced
- 4 cups vegetable broth (low-sodium)
- 2 tbsp fresh dill, chopped
- 1 cup almond milk (unsweetened)
- Salt (limited) and black pepper to taste
- Dill fronds for garnish

Directions:

1. Preheat oven to 400°F (200°C). Toss beets in 1 tbsp olive oil and spread on a baking sheet. Roast for 30 minutes or until tender.
2. The remaining olive oil should be heated in a big pot over medium heat. Add onions and garlic; sauté until translucent.
3. Add roasted beets and vegetable broth to the pool.
4. Boil for a few minutes, then boil the heat and simmer for ten.
5. Until the soup is creamy, purée it using an immersion blender.
6. Add fresh dill and almond milk after that. Add a little salt and pepper for seasoning.
7. Garnish with dill fronds before serving.

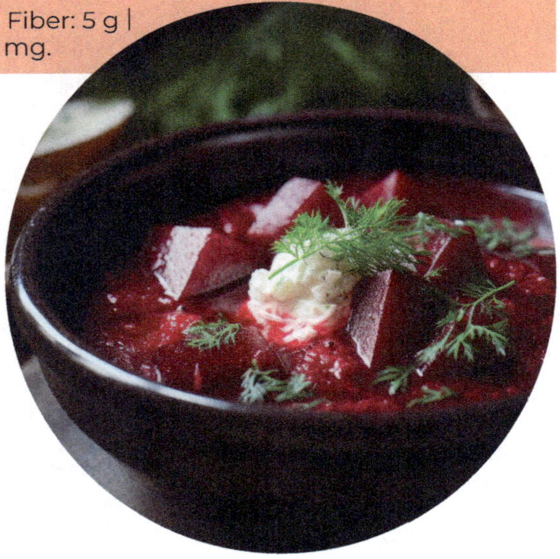

Heart-Healthy Benefits: *Nitrate, a substance included in beets, can improve blood flow and lower blood pressure. They also contain fiber, which supports cardiovascular health. Dill offers antioxidant properties.*

TURMERIC INFUSED POTATO LEEK SOUP

Calories: 220 kCal | Protein: 4 g | Carbohydrates: 40 g | Sugar: 5 g | Fat: 7 g | Fiber: 5 g | Cholesterol: 0 mg | Sodium: 150 mg | Phosphorus: 80 mg | Potassium: 800 mg.

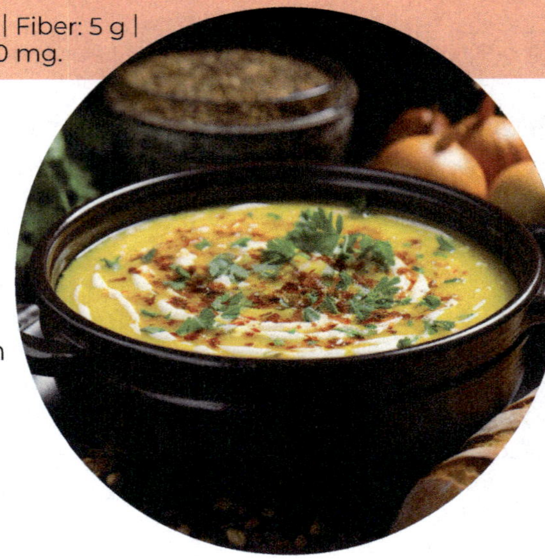

15 min | 25 min | 4

Ingredients:

- 3 tbsp olive oil
- Two leeks, white and light green parts only, cleaned and sliced
- Three cloves garlic, minced
- 4 cups potatoes, peeled and diced
- 5 cups vegetable broth (low-sodium)
- 1 tsp turmeric powder
- Salt (limited) and black pepper to taste
- Fresh parsley for garnish

Directions:

1. Olive oil is heated in a sizable pot over a medium flame. Add leeks and sauté until soft, about 5 minutes.
2. Add garlic and continue to sauté for another minute.
3. Incorporate potatoes, then pour in the vegetable broth.
4. Bring the mixture to a boil. Once boiling, reduce the heat and simmer until the potatoes are tender approximately 15 minutes.
5. Stir in the turmeric powder.
6. Use an immersion blender to puree the soup to the desired smoothness.
7. Season with a bit of salt and pepper. Garnish with fresh parsley before serving.

Heart-Healthy Benefits: *Curcumin, an anti-inflammatory and antioxidant substance good for heart health, is a component of turmeric. Potassium, which can help control blood pressure, is abundant in potatoes. Due to their flavonoid content, leeks, part of the allium family, have been linked to improved heart health.*

TUSCAN WHITE BEAN & ROSEMARY SOUP

Calories: 200 kCal | Protein: 10 g | Carbohydrates: 36 g | Sugar: 2 g | Fat: 4 g | Fiber: 8 g | Cholesterol: 0 mg | Sodium: 170 mg | Phosphorus: 120 mg | Potassium: 730 mg.

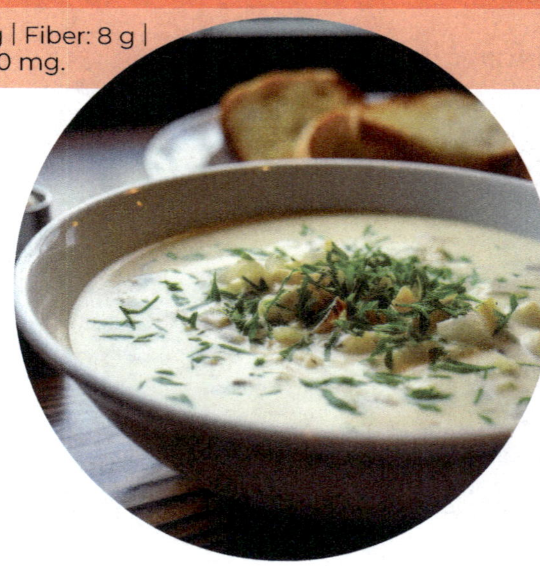

10 min | 25 min | 6

Ingredients:

- 2 tbsp olive oil
- One onion, finely chopped
- Three cloves garlic, minced
- 4 cups vegetable broth (low-sodium)
- Two cans (15 oz each) of white beans, drained and rinsed
- 2 tsp fresh rosemary, finely chopped
- Salt (limited) and black pepper to taste
- Grated lemon zest for garnish

Directions:

1. In a large pot, heat olive oil over medium heat. Add onions and sauté until translucent, then add garlic and continue to sauté for another minute.
2. Add the white beans, rosemary, and vegetable broth. Bring to a boil.
3. Reduce heat and simmer for 20 minutes.
4. Use an immersion blender to blend half of the soup, leaving some beans whole for texture.
5. Season with a pinch of salt and black pepper.
6. Garnish with grated lemon zest before serving.

Heart-Healthy Benefits: *A fantastic source of fiber that is good for the heart is found in white beans. Rosemary contains antioxidant and anti-inflammatory compounds. There are many heart-healthy monounsaturated fats in olive oil.*

ROASTED CAULIFLOWER & NUTMEG SOUP

Calories: 170 kCal | Protein: 4 g | Carbohydrates: 20 g | Sugar: 6 g | Fat: 10 g | Fiber: 5 g | Cholesterol: 0 mg | Sodium: 180 mg | Phosphorus: 100 mg | Potassium: 500 mg.

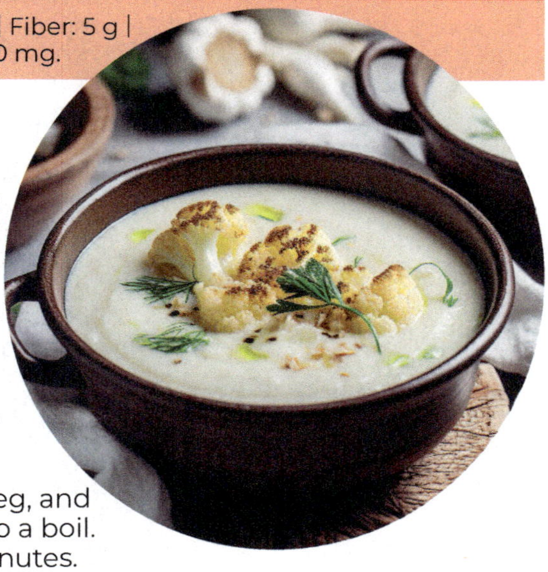

10 min | 40 min | 4

INGREDIENTS:

- One large head of cauliflower, cut into florets
- 3 tbsp olive oil, divided
- One onion, diced
- Three cloves garlic, minced
- 4 cups vegetable broth (low-sodium)
- 1/2 tsp freshly grated nutmeg
- Salt (limited) and black pepper to taste
- Fresh parsley for garnish

DIRECTIONS:

1. Preheat your oven to 425°F (220°C). Toss cauliflower florets in 2 tablespoons of olive oil and spread them on a baking sheet. Roast for 25-30 minutes or until golden and tender.
2. In a large pot, heat the remaining olive oil over medium heat. Add onions and sauté until translucent, then add garlic and continue to sauté for another minute.
3. Add the roasted cauliflower, nutmeg, and vegetable broth to the pot. Bring to a boil.
4. Reduce heat and simmer for 10 minutes.
5. Use an immersion blender to blend the soup until smooth. Season with a pinch of salt and black pepper.
6. Garnish with fresh parsley before serving.

Heart-Healthy Benefits: *Cauliflower is a cruciferous vegetable, which has been linked to a reduced risk of heart disease due to its high fiber and antioxidant content. Nutmeg adds depth of flavor and has potential anti-inflammatory properties. Olive oil, as mentioned, is a source of heart-friendly monounsaturated fats.*

SPINACH & FETA CREAM SOUP

Calories: 130 kCal | Protein: 5 g | Carbohydrates: 10 g | Sugar: 4 g | Fat: 8 g | Fiber: 2 g | Cholesterol: 15 mg | Sodium: 180 mg | Phosphorus: 90 mg | Potassium: 360 mg.

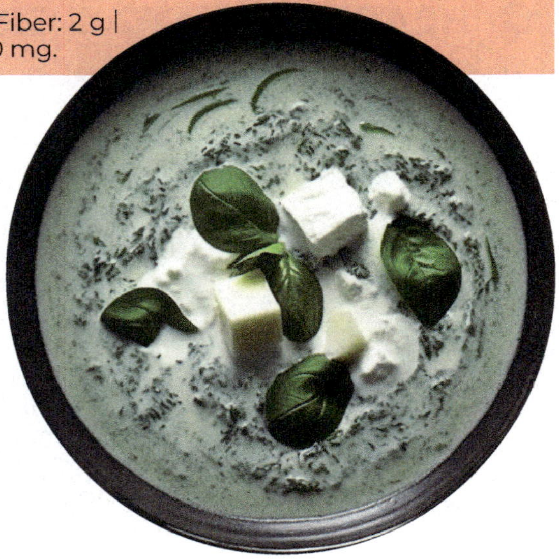

15 min | 45 min | 4

INGREDIENTS:

- 6 cups fresh spinach, washed and roughly chopped
- 1 tbsp olive oil
- One onion, finely chopped
- Two cloves garlic, minced
- 4 cups low-sodium vegetable broth
- 1 cup unsweetened almond milk
- 1/2 cup crumbled feta cheese (ensure a low-sodium variant)
- Freshly ground black pepper to taste
- A squeeze of lemon juice

DIRECTIONS:

1. In a large pot, heat olive oil over medium heat. Add onion and sauté until translucent.
2. Stir in garlic and cook for another 1-2 minutes.
3. Add spinach and sauté until wilted.
4. Pour in the vegetable broth and almond milk. Bring to a boil and let it simmer for about 10 minutes.
5. Remove from heat and blend the soup until smooth using an immersion blender.
6. Stir in crumbled feta cheese until it melts into the soup. Season with freshly ground black pepper and a squeeze of lemon juice.

Heart-Healthy Benefits: *Spinach is rich in vitamins, antioxidants, and dietary fiber, which can promote heart health. Feta cheese provides calcium without excessive fat, and when used in moderation and ensuring low-sodium variants, it can be a part of a heart-healthy diet. As previously noted, olive oil offers monounsaturated fats that benefit heart health.*

CREAMY ASPARAGUS & CHIVE SOUP

Calories: 90 kCal | Protein: 3 g | Carbohydrates: 12 g | Sugar: 5 g | Fat: 4 g | Fiber: 2 g | Cholesterol: 0 mg | Sodium: 150 mg | Phosphorus: 70 mg | Potassium: 340 mg.

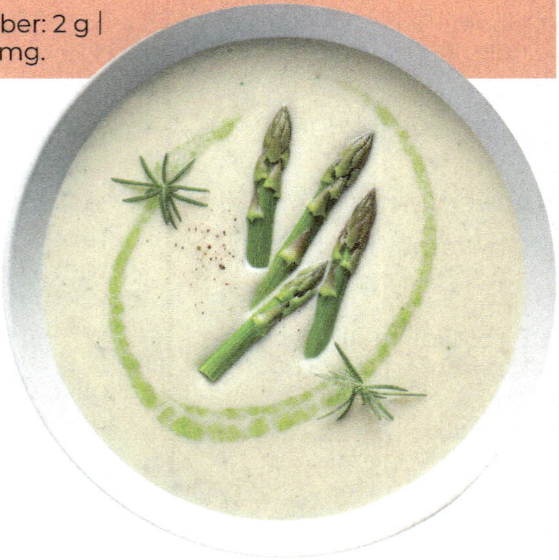

10 min | 25 min | 4

INGREDIENTS:

- One bunch of asparagus, trimmed and cut into 1-inch pieces
- 1 tbsp olive oil
- One onion, diced
- Two cloves garlic, minced
- 4 cups low-sodium vegetable broth
- 1/4 cup fresh chives, chopped, plus extra for garnish
- 1/2 cup unsweetened almond milk
- Freshly ground black pepper to taste

DIRECTIONS:

1. In a large pot, heat olive oil over medium heat. Add onions and sauté until translucent.
2. Stir in garlic and asparagus pieces. Cook for about 5 minutes.
3. Pour in the vegetable broth and bring the mixture to a boil. Reduce heat and simmer for 15 minutes or until the asparagus is tender.
4. Remove from heat and blend the soup until smooth using an immersion blender.
5. Stir in almond milk and chopped chives. Season with freshly ground black pepper.
6. Serve hot, garnished with extra chopped chives.

Heart-Healthy Benefits: *Asparagus is packed with nutrients, including fiber, vitamins A, C, E, and K, and chromium, a trace mineral that enhances the ability of insulin to transport glucose. It also contains a unique combination of anti-inflammatory nutrients, beneficial for heart health. Chives are related to garlic and onions and have similar heart-healthy benefits, including allicin, which can help reduce cholesterol and lower blood pressure.*

HEARTY POTATO & GREEN ONION SOUP

Calories: 210 kCal | Protein: 4 g | Carbohydrates: 40 g | Sugar: 3 g | Fat: 4 g | Fiber: 5 g | Cholesterol: 0 mg | Sodium: 130 mg | Phosphorus: 75 mg | Potassium: 800 mg.

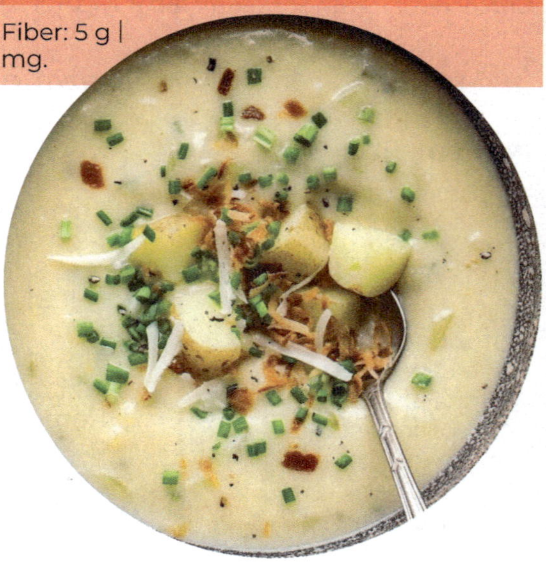

10 min | 30 min | 6

INGREDIENTS:

- Four large potatoes, peeled and diced
- 1 tbsp olive oil
- One bunch of green onions, chopped (separate white and green parts)
- Three cloves garlic, minced
- 5 cups low-sodium vegetable broth
- Freshly ground black pepper to taste
- Fresh parsley, chopped, for garnish

DIRECTIONS:

1. In a large pot, heat olive oil over medium heat. Add the white parts of the green onions and sauté until translucent.
2. Add garlic and stir for another minute.
3. Add diced potatoes and vegetable broth. Bring to a boil.
4. Reduce heat and simmer for about 20-25 minutes or until potatoes are tender.
5. Blend half the soup using an immersion blender, leaving some chunks for texture.
6. Stir in the green parts of the onions. Season with black pepper.
7. Serve hot, garnished with fresh parsley.

Heart-Healthy Benefits: *Potatoes are a good source of vitamin C, vitamin B6, and fiber when the skins are consumed. They're also rich in potassium, which can help lower blood pressure. Green onions, or scallions, are rich in antioxidants, which help reduce the risk of chronic diseases, including cardiovascular diseases.*

HERB-INFUSED VEGETABLE MEDLEY STEW

Calories: 150 kCal | Protein: 3 g | Carbohydrates: 25 g | Sugar: 7 g | Fat: 6 g | Fiber: 6 g | Cholesterol: 0 mg | Sodium: 120 mg | Phosphorus: 80 mg | Potassium: 450 mg.

15 min | 40 min | 4

INGREDIENTS:

- 2 tbsp olive oil
- One onion, chopped
- Two cloves garlic, minced
- Two carrots, sliced
- One zucchini, cubed
- One bell pepper, chopped
- 4 cups low-sodium vegetable broth
- One can (14 oz) diced tomatoes, no salt added
- 2 tsp dried Italian herb mix (basil, oregano, thyme, rosemary)
- Freshly ground black pepper to taste
- Fresh parsley, chopped, for garnish

DIRECTIONS:

1. In a large pot, heat olive oil over medium heat. Add onion and garlic, sautéing until translucent.
2. Add carrots, zucchini, and bell pepper. Cook for another 5 minutes, stirring occasionally.
3. Stir in the vegetable broth, diced tomatoes, and Italian herbs.
4. Bring to a boil, reduce heat, cover, and let simmer for 30 minutes.
5. Season with freshly ground black pepper.
6. Serve hot, garnished with fresh parsley.

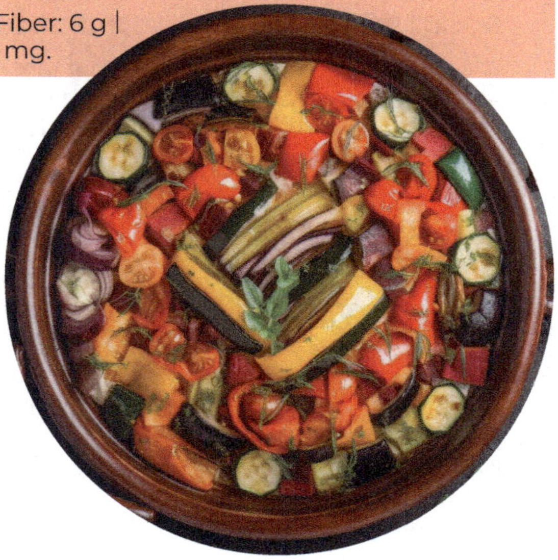

Heart-Healthy Benefits: *The combination of vegetables provides a wealth of nutrients, including dietary fiber, which helps reduce cholesterol. The Italian herbs are not just for flavor but also offer antioxidant properties. Tomatoes are especially beneficial for heart health due to their lycopene content, a potent antioxidant.*

SPICED CHICKPEA & SPINACH STEW

Calories: 190 kCal | Protein: 7 g | Carbohydrates: 28 g | Sugar: 4 g | Fat: 6 g | Fiber: 8 g | Cholesterol: 0 mg | Sodium: 150 mg | Phosphorus: 110 mg | Potassium: 500 mg.

15 min | 45 min | 6

INGREDIENTS:

- 2 tbsp olive oil
- One onion, diced
- Three cloves garlic, minced
- One can (14 oz) chickpeas, drained and rinsed
- 5 cups spinach, washed and roughly chopped
- 5 cups low-sodium vegetable broth
- 1 tsp ground cumin
- 1 tsp ground coriander
- 1/2 tsp smoked paprika
- Freshly ground black pepper to taste
- Lemon wedges for serving

DIRECTIONS:

1. Heat olive oil in a pot over medium heat. Add onion and garlic and sauté until soft.
2. Stir in the chickpeas, cumin, coriander, and smoked paprika, cooking for 2-3 minutes.
3. Add the vegetable broth and bring to a boil. Reduce heat and simmer for 20 minutes.
4. Stir in the spinach, cooking just until wilted.
5. Season with black pepper and serve hot with lemon wedges.

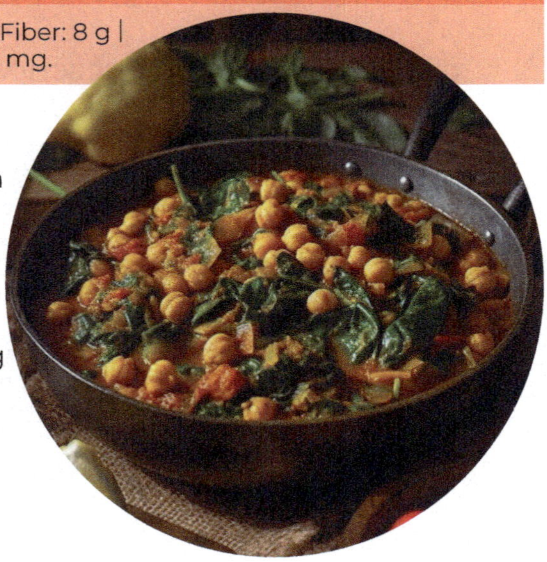

Heart-Healthy Benefits: *Chickpeas are a heart-healthy choice due to their fiber, potassium, and vitamin content. Spinach, rich in magnesium and nitrates, is known to help regulate blood pressure. The spices enhance flavor and bring in additional heart benefits - for instance, cumin can help improve cholesterol levels.*

TUSCAN WHITE BEAN & SPINACH STEW

Calories: 250 kCal | Protein: 11 g | Carbohydrates: 41 g | Sugar: 2 g | Fat: 6 g | Fiber: 10 g | Cholesterol: 0 mg | Sodium: 140 mg | Phosphorus: 140 mg | Potassium: 650 mg.

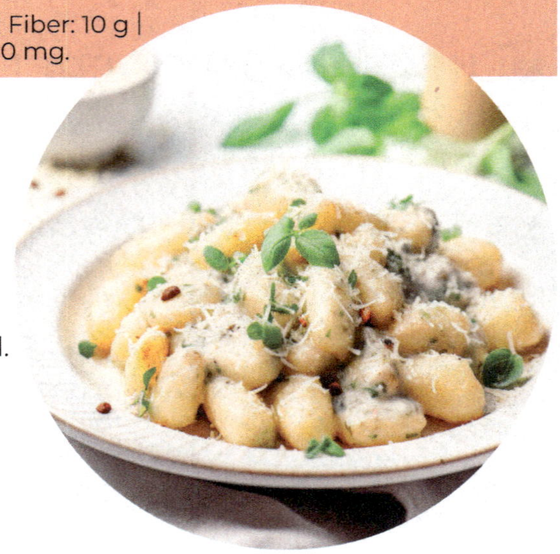

10 min | 30 min | 4

INGREDIENTS:

- Two cans (14 oz each) of white beans, drained and rinsed
- 4 cups fresh spinach, washed and roughly chopped
- One onion, diced
- Two cloves garlic, minced
- 2 tbsp olive oil
- 4 cups low-sodium vegetable broth
- 1 tsp dried rosemary
- Freshly ground black pepper to taste
- Grated zest of 1 lemon

DIRECTIONS:

1. In a large pot, heat the olive oil. Add onion and garlic and sauté until translucent.
2. Stir in white beans and vegetable broth. Bring to a simmer.
3. Add spinach and rosemary, cooking until the spinach is wilted.
4. Season with black pepper and lemon zest.
5. Serve hot.

Heart-Healthy Benefits: *White beans are a great source of fiber and protein, making them beneficial for heart health. As mentioned, spinach offers magnesium and nitrates to help regulate blood pressure. Lemon zest gives a refreshing twist and contains flavonoids, which might help to reduce inflammation and improve blood vessel function.*

HEARTY MUSHROOM & PEARL BARLEY STEW

Calories: 270 kCal | Protein: 8 g | Carbohydrates: 51 g | Sugar: 3 g | Fat: 7 g | Fiber: 9 g | Cholesterol: 0 mg | Sodium: 115 mg | Phosphorus: 120 mg | Potassium: 400 mg.

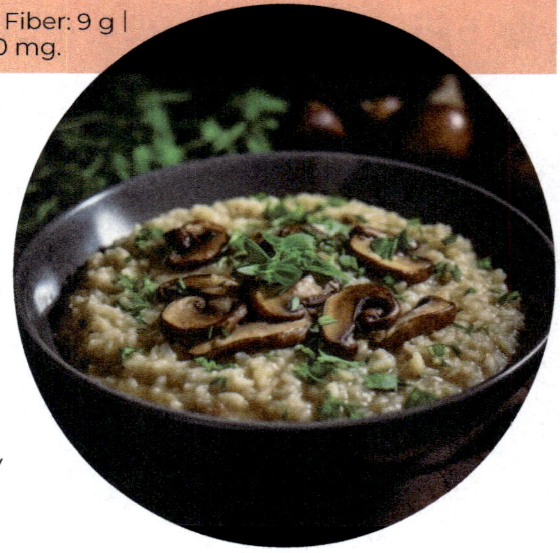

15 min | 50 min | 4

INGREDIENTS:

- 1 cup pearl barley, rinsed
- 2 cups sliced mixed mushrooms (e.g., cremini, shiitake, oyster)
- One onion, diced
- Two cloves garlic, minced
- 2 tbsp olive oil
- 5 cups low-sodium vegetable broth
- 1 tsp dried thyme
- Freshly ground black pepper to taste
- Fresh parsley, chopped for garnish

DIRECTIONS:

1. In a large pot, heat the olive oil over medium heat. Add the onion and garlic, and sauté until translucent.
2. Stir in mushrooms and cook until they begin to release their juices.
3. Add pearl barley, thyme, and vegetable broth to the pot.
4. Bring the mixture to a boil, then reduce to a simmer. Cover and cook for 45 minutes or until barley is tender.
5. Season with freshly ground black pepper.
6. Serve hot, garnished with fresh parsley.

Heart-Healthy Benefits: *Mushrooms are low in calories and sodium, yet they provide essential nutrients, including selenium, potassium, riboflavin, niacin, and vitamin D, which benefit heart health. Pearl barley is rich in soluble fiber and can help reduce blood cholesterol levels.*

FIERY TOMATO & QUINOA STEW

Calories: 160 kCal | Protein: 6 g | Carbohydrates: 25 g | Sugar: 3 g | Fat: 4 g | Fiber: 3 g | Cholesterol: 0 mg | Sodium: 200 mg | Phosphorus: 45 mg | Potassium: 350 mg.

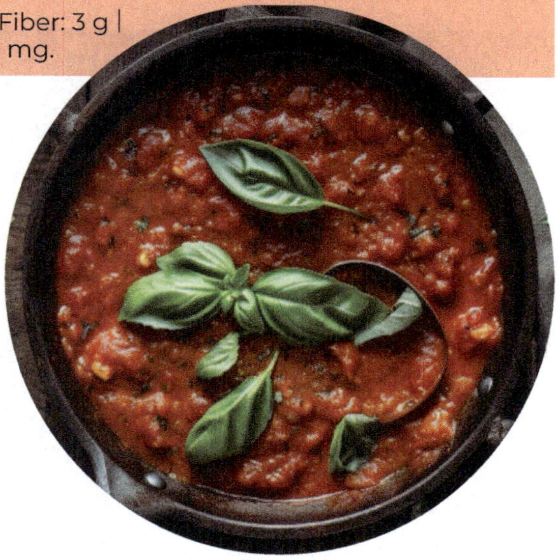

15 min | 25 min | 4

INGREDIENTS:

- 1 cup cooked quinoa
- 2 cups tomatoes, diced
- One red chili pepper deseeded and finely chopped
- Two cloves garlic, minced
- 3 cups low-sodium vegetable broth
- 1 tbsp olive oil
- 1 tsp paprika
- 1/2 tsp cayenne pepper (adjust to preference)
- Fresh cilantro for garnish

DIRECTIONS:

1. In a large pot, heat the olive oil over medium heat. Add minced garlic and chopped chili pepper, sautéing until aromatic.
2. Stir in tomatoes and season with paprika and cayenne.
3. Pour in vegetable broth and bring the mixture to a boil.
4. Once boiling, add in cooked quinoa and let simmer for 10-15 minutes, allowing flavors to meld.
5. Serve hot, garnishing with fresh cilantro.

Heart-Healthy Benefits: *It can enhance heart health and lower blood sugar levels. The antioxidant lycopene, which has been linked to a lower risk of heart disease, and the heart-healthy potassium found in tomatoes are both abundant in tomatoes.*

HEARTY BEET & CARROT STEW

Calories: 110 kCal | Protein: 3 g | Carbohydrates: 20 g | Sugar: 8 g | Fat: 3 g | Fiber: 4 g | Cholesterol: 0 mg | Sodium: 190 mg | Phosphorus: 40 mg | Potassium: 400 mg.

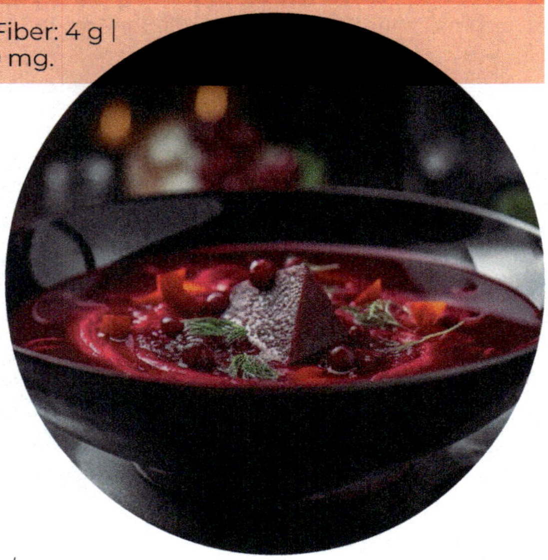

20 min | 35 min | 4

INGREDIENTS:

- Two medium-sized beets, peeled and diced
- Two large carrots, sliced
- One onion, chopped
- 3 cups low-sodium vegetable broth
- 1 tbsp olive oil
- 1 tsp thyme
- Salt and pepper to taste
- Fresh parsley for garnish

DIRECTIONS:

1. Olive oil is heated in a pot over a medium flame. Add onions and sauté until translucent.
2. Stir in beets and carrots, cooking for a few minutes.
3. Add vegetable broth, thyme, salt, and pepper. Bring to a boil.
4. Reduce heat to low and simmer for 25-30 minutes or until beets and carrots are tender.
5. Garnish with fresh parsley before serving.

Heart-Healthy Benefits: *It can enhance heart health and lower blood sugar levels. The antioxidant lycopene, which has been linked to a lower risk of heart disease, and the heart-healthy potassium found in tomatoes are both abundant in tomatoes.*

NOTES

Poultry Recipes

LEMON HERB GRILLED CHICKEN BREASTS

Calories: 220 kCal | Protein: 28 g | Carbohydrates: 5 g | Sugar: 2 g | Fat: 10 g | Fiber: 1 g | Cholesterol: 70 mg | Sodium: 150 mg | Phosphorus: 30 mg | Potassium: 220 mg.

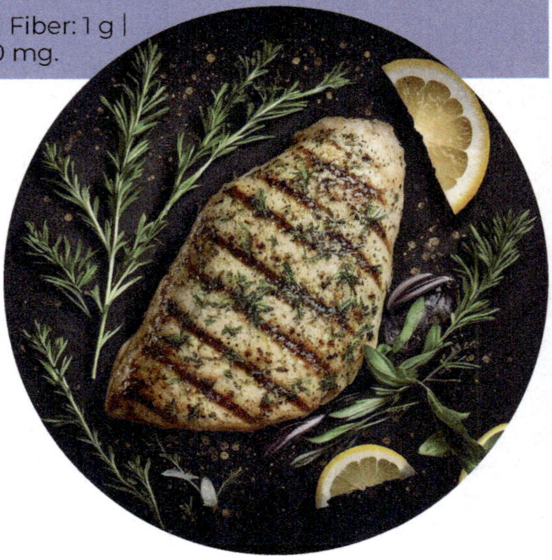

15 min | 15 min | 4

Ingredients:

- Four boneless, skinless chicken breasts
- Two lemons, zested and juiced
- 3 tbsp olive oil
- Two cloves garlic, minced
- 1 tbsp fresh rosemary, finely chopped
- Salt (be mindful of the amount) and black pepper to taste

Directions:

1. Whisk together lemon zest, lemon juice, olive oil, garlic, rosemary, salt, and pepper in a bowl.
2. Marinate chicken breasts in the mixture for at least 1 hour.
3. Preheat the grill to medium-high. Grill chicken for 6-7 minutes on each side or until fully cooked.
4. Let rest for 5 minutes before serving.

Heart-Healthy Benefits: *Chicken breasts provide lean protein, which supports heart health. Lemons contain vitamin C, essential for maintaining the health of blood vessels. There are many heart-healthy monounsaturated fats in olive oil.*

ROSEMARY INFUSED TURKEY TENDERLOIN

Calories: 210 kCal | Protein: 30 g | Carbohydrates: 4 g | Sugar: 1 g | Fat: 9 g | Fiber: 1 g | Cholesterol: 60 mg | Sodium: 130 mg | Phosphorus: 25 mg | Potassium: 210 mg.

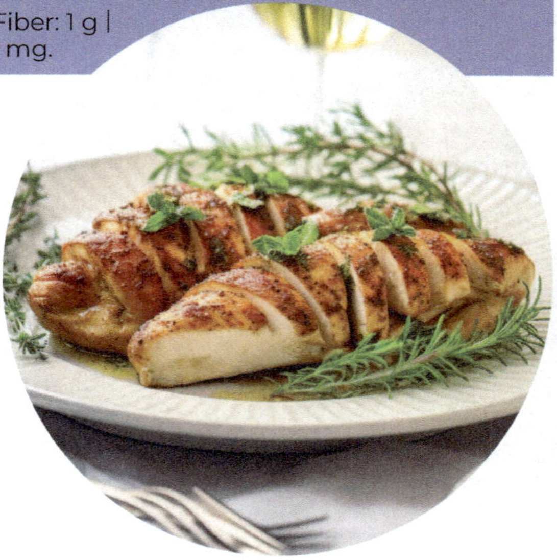

10 min | 25 min | 4

Ingredients:

- Two turkey tenderloins (about 1 lb total)
- 2 tbsp fresh rosemary, finely chopped
- Two cloves garlic, minced
- 3 tbsp olive oil
- One lemon, zested and juiced
- Salt (be mindful of the amount) and black pepper to taste

Directions:

1. Preheat oven to 375°F (190°C).
2. Mix rosemary, garlic, olive oil, lemon zest, lemon juice, salt, and pepper in a bowl. Rub this mixture over the turkey tenderloins.
3. Place tenderloins in a roasting pan. Bake for 20-25 minutes or until fully cooked.
4. Let rest for 5 minutes before slicing and serving.

Heart-Healthy Benefits: *Turkey is a lean source of protein. Rosemary contains antioxidants that support heart health.*

NOTES

MEDITERRANEAN CHICKEN SKEWERS

Calories: 200 kCal | Protein: 25 g | Carbohydrates: 6 g | Sugar: 3 g | Fat: 10 g | Fiber: 2 g | Cholesterol: 65 mg | Sodium: 140 mg | Phosphorus: 20 mg | Potassium: 300 mg.

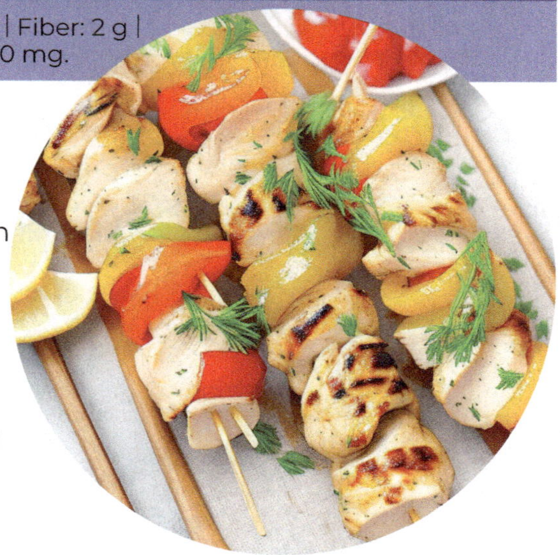

20 min (plus marination) | 12 min | 4

Ingredients:

- Two boneless, skinless chicken breasts, cubed
- One red bell pepper, cubed
- One zucchini, sliced
- 1/4 cup olive oil
- One lemon, zested and juiced
- Two cloves garlic, minced
- 1 tsp dried oregano
- Salt (be mindful of the amount) and black pepper to taste

Directions:

1. Mix olive oil, lemon zest, lemon juice, garlic, oregano, salt, and pepper in a bowl. Marinate chicken cubes in this mixture for at least 2 hours.
2. Preheat grill to medium-high. Thread chicken, bell pepper, and zucchini onto skewers.
3. Grill skewers on each side for 5-6 minutes or until chicken is cooked through.
4. Serve immediately.

Heart-Healthy Benefits: *Chicken provides lean protein. Red bell peppers are rich in antioxidants and vitamin C, which benefit heart health. Zucchini offers dietary fiber, which is beneficial for heart health.*

HONEY MUSTARD GLAZED CHICKEN THIGHS

Calories: 230 kCal | Protein: 22 g | Carbohydrates: 12 g | Sugar: 10 g | Fat: 10 g | Fiber: 0 g | Cholesterol: 85 mg | Sodium: 160 mg | Phosphorus: 15 mg | Potassium: 240 mg.

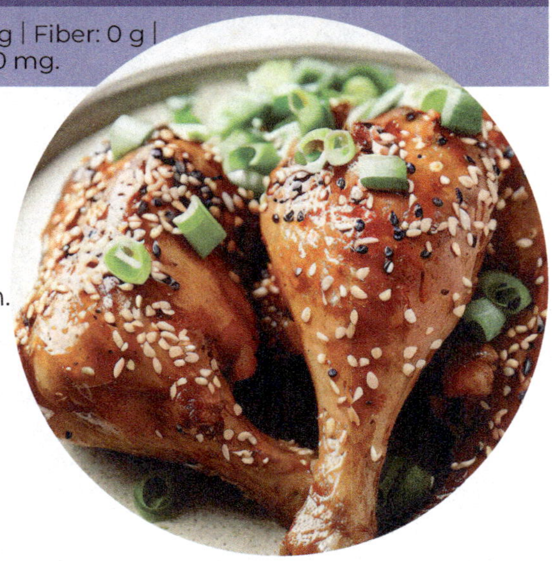

10 min | 20 min | 4

Ingredients:

- Four boneless, skinless chicken thighs
- 2 tbsp honey
- 2 tbsp Dijon mustard
- 2 tbsp olive oil
- One clove of garlic, minced
- Salt (be mindful of the amount) and black pepper to taste

Directions:

1. Preheat oven to 400°F (200°C).
2. Mix honey, mustard, olive oil, garlic, salt, and pepper in a bowl.
3. Coat chicken thighs with the mixture and place in a baking dish.
4. Bake for 20 minutes or until fully cooked, basting occasionally with the sauce.
5. Serve immediately.

Heart-Healthy Benefits: *Chicken thighs provide lean protein. Honey contains antioxidants that support heart health. Mustard and olive oil contain healthy fats that can help lower harmful cholesterol levels.*

NOTES

TARRAGON & ORANGE ROASTED CHICKEN

Calories: 220 kCal | Protein: 28 g | Carbohydrates: 10 g | Sugar: 8 g | Fat: 10 g | Fiber: 1 g | Cholesterol: 70 mg | Sodium: 150 mg | Phosphorus: 25 mg | Potassium: 290 mg.

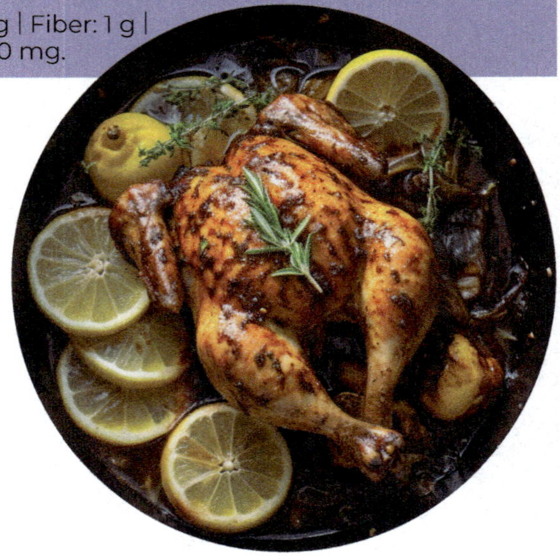

15 min | 35 min | 4

INGREDIENTS:

- Four boneless, skinless chicken breasts
- Two oranges, zested and juiced
- 2 tbsp fresh tarragon, finely chopped
- 3 tbsp olive oil
- Two cloves garlic, minced
- Salt (be mindful of the amount) and black pepper to taste

DIRECTIONS:

1. Preheat oven to 375°F (190°C).
2. Mix orange zest, juice, tarragon, olive oil, garlic, salt, and pepper in a bowl.
3. Place chicken in a roasting pan and pour the mixture over it.
4. Bake for 30-35 minutes or until chicken is fully cooked, basting occasionally with the sauce.
5. Let rest for 5 minutes before serving.

Heart-Healthy Benefits: *Chicken breasts provide lean protein. Oranges are a good fiber and vitamin C source suitable for the heart. Antioxidants in tarragon are good for the soul.*

SESAME GINGER CHICKEN LETTUCE WRAPS

Calories: 180 kCal | Protein: 25 g | Carbohydrates: 8 g | Sugar: 4 g | Fat: 5 g | Fiber: 2 g | Cholesterol: 65 mg | Sodium: 180 mg | Phosphorus: 40 mg | Potassium: 320 mg.

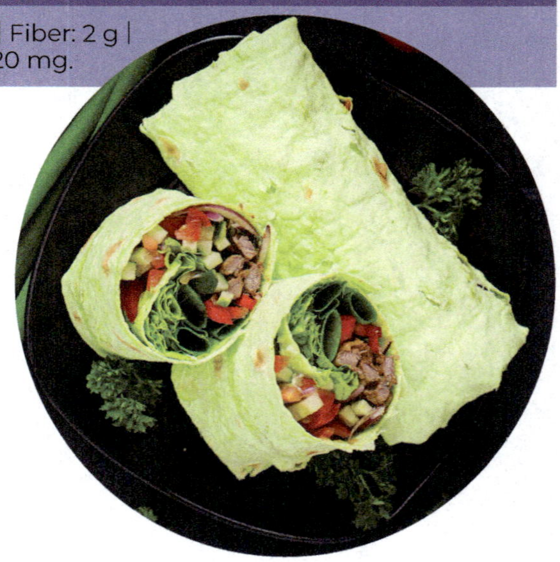

20 min | 15 min | 4

INGREDIENTS:

- Two boneless, skinless chicken breasts, finely chopped
- 1 tbsp sesame oil
- 2 tbsp fresh ginger, grated
- Two garlic cloves, minced
- 1/4 cup low-sodium soy sauce
- 1/2 cup diced bell peppers (any color)
- 1/2 cup diced cucumbers
- 1/4 cup chopped green onions
- 8-12 lettuce leaves (like Romaine or Butterhead)
- 1 tbsp toasted sesame seeds

DIRECTIONS:

1. Heat sesame oil in a skillet over medium heat. Add ginger and garlic and sauté for 2 minutes.
2. Add the finely chopped chicken to the skillet and cook until no longer pink.
3. Pour in the low-sodium soy sauce and stir for 2-3 minutes.
4. Add bell peppers and cucumbers, cooking just until slightly tender.
5. Serve the chicken mixture in lettuce leaves, garnished with green onions and sesame seeds.

Heart-Healthy Benefits: *Chicken offers lean protein, while sesame seeds and oil provide heart-healthy fats. Ginger supports circulation and has anti-inflammatory properties. Lettuce is low-calorie and adds crunch without added sodium or fat.*

CILANTRO LIME TURKEY BURGERS

Calories: 190 kCal | Protein: 30 g | Carbohydrates: 2 g | Sugar: 1 g | Fat: 8 g | Fiber: 0 g | Cholesterol: 75 mg | Sodium: 130 mg | Phosphorus: 20 mg | Potassium: 250 mg.

15 min | 35 min | 4

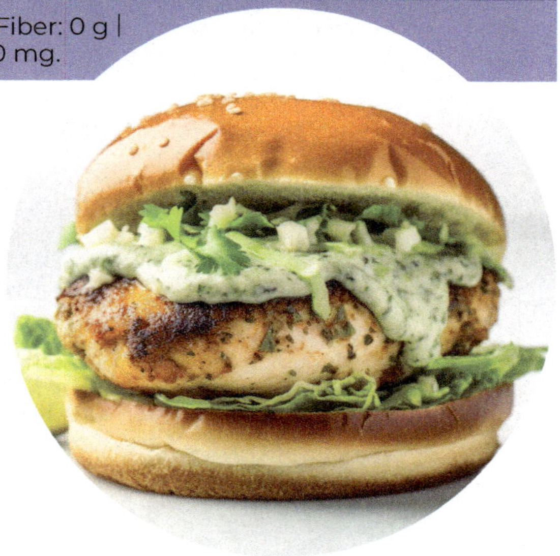

INGREDIENTS:

- 1 lb ground turkey (lean)
- 2 tbsp fresh cilantro, finely chopped
- Zest and juice of 1 lime
- One garlic clove, minced
- 1/2 tsp ground cumin
- Salt (be mindful of the amount) and black pepper to taste
- Four whole-grain buns (optional)

DIRECTIONS:

1. Combine ground turkey, cilantro, zest, lime juice, garlic, cumin, salt, and pepper in a mixing bowl.
2. Form into four even patties.
3. Preheat the grill or stovetop pan to medium-high heat. Cook patties on each side for 6-7 minutes or until fully cooked.
4. Serve on whole grain buns if desired, or eat as is for a lower-carb option.

Heart-Healthy Benefits: *Ground turkey is a heart-healthy protein alternative to beef that is leaner. Cilantro has antioxidants, and lime provides vitamin C. Cumin can help digestion and contains beneficial antioxidants.*

GARLIC & HERB BAKED TURKEY MEATBALLS

Calories: 210 kCal | Protein: 28 g | Carbohydrates: 6 g | Sugar: 1 g | Fat: 8 g | Fiber: 1 g | Cholesterol: 85 mg | Sodium: 160 mg | Phosphorus: 25 mg | Potassium: 280 mg.

15 min | 20 min | 4

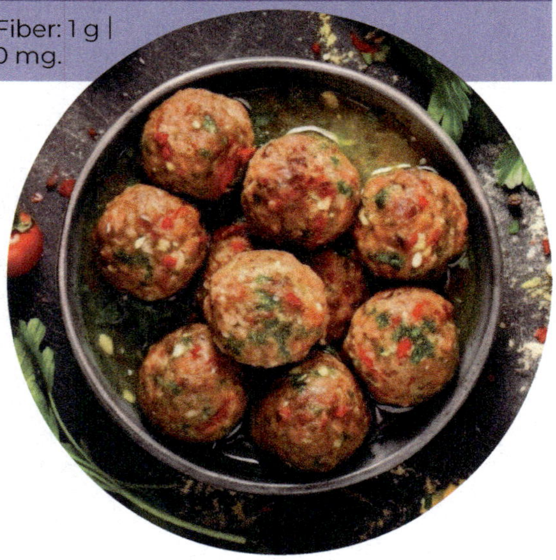

INGREDIENTS:

- 1 lb lean ground turkey
- Two garlic cloves, minced
- 2 tbsp fresh parsley, chopped
- 1 tbsp fresh basil, chopped
- 1/4 cup breadcrumbs (whole grain)
- One egg
- Salt (be mindful of the amount) and black pepper to taste

DIRECTIONS:

1. Preheat oven to 400°F (200°C).
2. In a bowl, combine all ingredients and mix until well combined.
3. Form into meatballs and place on a lined baking sheet.
4. Bake for 18-20 minutes or until fully cooked.

Heart-Healthy Benefits: *Without the saturated fat in red meat, lean ground turkey is a fantastic source of protein. Blood pressure and cholesterol can both be reduced with garlic. Parsley and basil provide vitamins and minerals that support heart health.*

NOTES

SPICED MAPLE TURKEY SAUSAGES

Calories: 180 kCal | Protein: 22 g | Carbohydrates: 5 g | Sugar: 4 g | Fat: 8 g | Fiber: 0 g | Cholesterol: 60 mg | Sodium: 160 mg | Phosphorus: 28 mg | Potassium: 290 mg.

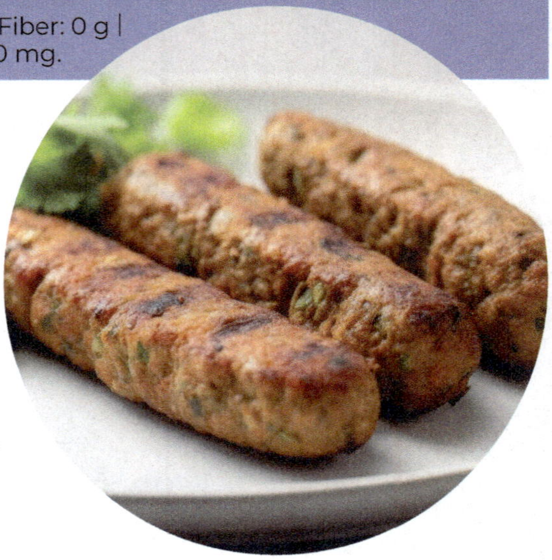

15 min | 15 min | 6

INGREDIENTS:

- 1 lb ground turkey
- 2 tbsp pure maple syrup
- 1 tsp smoked paprika
- 1/2 tsp ground cumin
- 1/4 tsp cayenne pepper (optional for heat)
- 1 tbsp olive oil
- Salt (be mindful of the amount)

DIRECTIONS:

1. Combine ground turkey, maple syrup, smoked paprika, cumin, and cayenne pepper in a mixing bowl. Mix until all ingredients are well integrated.
2. Form the mixture into small sausage shapes.
3. Heat olive oil in a skillet over medium heat.
4. Cook the sausages for 5-6 minutes on each side or until fully cooked.
5. Lightly season with salt before serving.

Heart-Healthy Benefits: *Turkey is a lean protein that aids heart muscle functionality. Maple syrup provides a natural, sweet touch without refined sugars. Spices add flavors and contain various health benefits; cumin can aid digestion and metabolism.*

TUSCAN HERB CHICKEN & VEGETABLE ROAST

Calories: 240 kCal | Protein: 28 g | Carbohydrates: 10 g | Sugar: 4 g | Fat: 10 g | Fiber: 2 g | Cholesterol: 95 mg | Sodium: 220 mg | Phosphorus: 40 mg | Potassium: 340 mg.

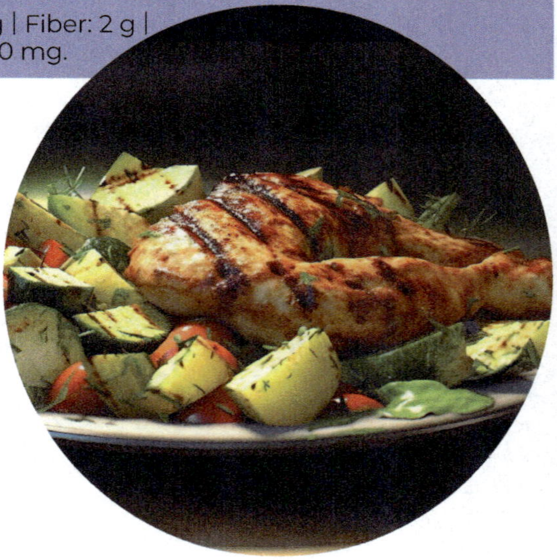

20 min | 40 min | 6

INGREDIENTS:

- 1.5 lbs boneless, skinless chicken thighs
- One zucchini, sliced
- One bell pepper, chopped
- One onion, chopped
- 2 tbsp olive oil
- 1 tbsp each of dried basil, oregano, and rosemary
- Salt (be mindful of the amount) and black pepper to taste

DIRECTIONS:

6. Preheat oven to 375°F (190°C).
7. Toss chicken and vegetables with olive oil, herbs, salt, and pepper in a large mixing bowl.
8. Spread the chicken and vegetable mixture on a large baking sheet or roasting pan.
9. Roast in the preheated oven for about 35-40 minutes or until chicken is cooked through and vegetables are tender.
10. Allow to rest for a few minutes before serving.

Heart-Healthy Benefits: *Zucchini, bell pepper, and onions are rich in vitamins and fiber, promoting heart health. The blend of herbs adds flavor and has some health advantages, including antioxidant and anti-inflammatory qualities.*

NOTES

MINT & GARLIC ROASTED CHICKEN QUARTERS

Calories: 310 kCal | Protein: 25 g | Carbohydrates: 4 g | Sugar: 1 g | Fat: 21 g | Fiber: 1 g | Cholesterol: 110 mg | Sodium: 200 mg | Phosphorus: 29 mg | Potassium: 290 mg.

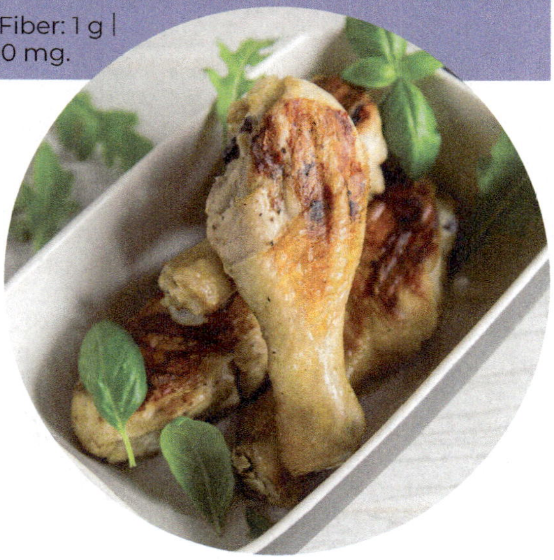

20 min | 40 min | 4

INGREDIENTS:

- Four chicken leg quarters
- 2 tbsp fresh mint leaves, finely chopped
- Three cloves garlic, minced
- 2 tbsp olive oil
- Zest and juice of 1 lemon
- Salt (be mindful of the amount) and freshly ground black pepper

DIRECTIONS:

1. Preheat oven to 400°F (200°C).
2. Mix mint, garlic, olive oil, lemon zest, and juice in a bowl.
3. Arrange chicken quarters on a baking tray, skin side up. Brush them generously with the mint-garlic mixture.
4. Season lightly with salt and pepper, then roast in the oven for about 35-40 minutes or until the chicken is golden brown and fully cooked.
5. Serve warm with steamed vegetables or a light salad.

Heart-Healthy Benefits: *Mint has antioxidants that can help reduce oxidative stress. Garlic has been known to offer many health benefits, including lowering blood pressure and cholesterol. Lemon provides vitamin C, which can support blood vessel function.*

MEAT (PORK, BEEF) RECIPES

HERB-CRUSTED PORK LOIN ROAST

Calories: 240 kCal | Protein: 30 g | Carbohydrates: 0 g | Sugar: 0 g | Fat: 11 g | Fiber: 0 g | Cholesterol: 75 mg | Sodium: 330 mg | Phosphorus: 250 mg | Potassium: 380 mg.

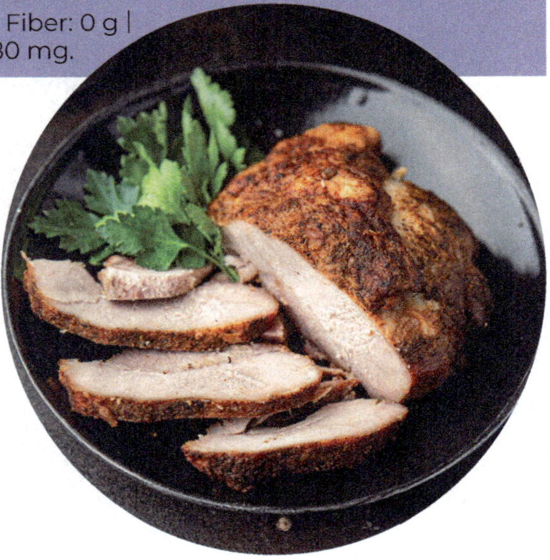

15 min | 45 min | 4

INGREDIENTS:

- One pork loin roast (about 2 lbs)
- 2 tbsp olive oil
- Two garlic cloves, minced
- 1 tsp dried rosemary
- 1 tsp dried thyme
- 1/2 tsp salt (ensure low sodium)
- 1/4 tsp black pepper

DIRECTIONS:

1. Preheat the oven to 375°F (190°C).
2. Mix olive oil, garlic, rosemary, thyme, salt, and pepper in a small bowl.
3. Rub the mixture over the pork loin roast, ensuring it's coated evenly.
4. Place the roast in a baking dish.
5. Bake in the oven for about 45 minutes or until the internal temperature reaches 145°F (62°C).
6. Remove from oven and let it rest for 10 minutes before slicing.

Heart-Healthy Benefits: *Monounsaturated fats, abundant in olive oil and can lower LDL (harmful) cholesterol levels, are beneficial. The herbs add flavor and possess antioxidant properties functional for heart health.*

ROSEMARY GARLIC BEEF SKEWERS

Calories: 220 kCal | Protein: 26 g | Carbohydrates: 1 g | Sugar: 0 g | Fat: 13 g | Fiber: 0 g | Cholesterol: 70 mg | Sodium: 200 mg | Phosphorus: 260 mg | Potassium: 340 mg.

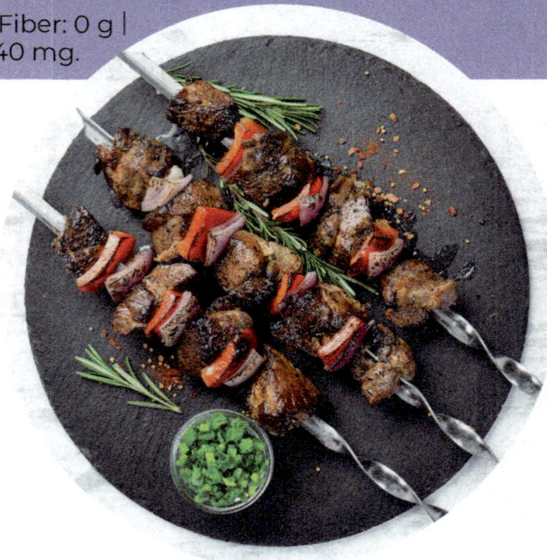

20 min (plus marination) | 8 min | 4

INGREDIENTS:

- 1 lb beef sirloin, cut into 1-inch cubes
- Three garlic cloves, minced
- 2 tbsp olive oil
- 1 tbsp fresh rosemary, finely chopped
- Salt (ensure low sodium) and pepper to taste

DIRECTIONS:

1. Combine garlic, olive oil, rosemary, salt, and pepper in a mixing bowl. Add beef cubes and toss to coat. Marinate for at least 2 hours in the refrigerator.
2. Preheat the grill to medium-high heat.
3. Thread the beef cubes onto skewers.
4. Grill the skewers for about 4 minutes on each side or until desired doneness is achieved.
5. Remove from grill and serve immediately.

Heart-Healthy Benefits: *Sirloin is a lean cut of beef, reducing saturated fat intake. Rosemary and garlic provide flavor and contain antioxidants that can help improve heart health.*

SPICED PORK & VEGETABLE STIR-FRY

Calories: 220 kCal | Protein: 28 g | Carbohydrates: 8 g | Sugar: 4 g | Fat: 8 g | Fiber: 2 g | Cholesterol: 70 mg | Sodium: 290 mg | Phosphorus: 240 mg | Potassium: 460 mg.

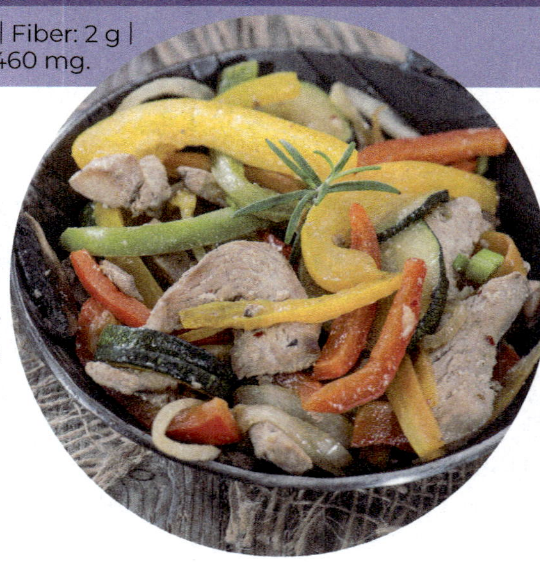

15 min | 12 min | 4

INGREDIENTS:

- 1 lb pork loin, thinly sliced
- One bell pepper, sliced
- One zucchini, sliced
- One carrot, julienned
- 3 tbsp low-sodium soy sauce
- 1 tbsp sesame oil
- 1 tsp ginger, minced
- One garlic clove, minced
- 1/2 tsp red pepper flakes

DIRECTIONS:

6. Warm the sesame oil over medium-high heat in a wok or sizable skillet. Add pork slices and cook until browned. Remove and set aside.
7. Add ginger, garlic, and red pepper flakes in the same wok. Sauté for a minute.
8. Add bell pepper, zucchini, and carrot. Stir-fry for about 4 minutes until vegetables are tender.
9. Return the pork to the wok, add low-sodium soy sauce, and stir well. Cook for another 3 minutes.
10. Serve immediately.

Heart-Healthy Benefits: *Lean pork and a variety of vegetables provide essential nutrients without excessive fats. Soy sauce adds flavor without much sodium, while ginger and garlic have anti-inflammatory properties beneficial for cardiovascular health.*

NOTES

TENDER BEEF MEDALLIONS WITH HERBED BUTTER

Calories: 250 kCal | Protein: 30 g | Carbohydrates: 1 g | Sugar: 0 g | Fat: 14 g | Fiber: 0 g | Cholesterol: 85 mg | Sodium: 230 mg | Phosphorus: 290 mg | Potassium: 370 mg.

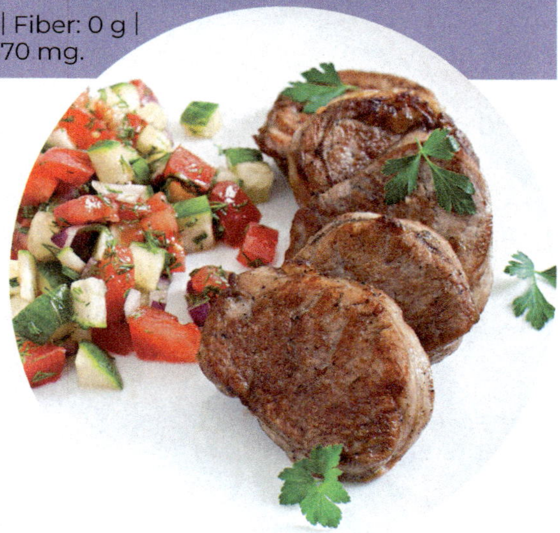

20 min | 8 min | 4

Ingredients:

- Four beef medallions (about 5 oz each)
- Salt (ensure low sodium) and pepper to taste

For Herbed Butter:

- 2 tbsp olive oil-based margarine
- 1 tbsp fresh parsley, finely chopped
- 1 tsp fresh chives, finely chopped
- One garlic clove, minced

Directions:

1. For the herbed butter: In a small bowl, mix margarine, parsley, chives, and garlic until well combined. Set aside.
2. Preheat the grill to medium-high heat.
3. Season beef medallions with salt and pepper.
4. Grill for 4-5 minutes on each side until the desired doneness is achieved.
5. Once off the grill, top each medallion with a dollop of herbed butter.

Heart-Healthy Benefits: *Beef medallions are a lean cut and provide high-quality protein. Olive oil-based margarine is a heart-healthy alternative to butter, and fresh herbs add flavor without sodium.*

MUSTARD GLAZED PORK CHOPS

Calories: 240 kCal | Protein: 28 g | Carbohydrates: 5 g | Sugar: 4 g | Fat: 11 g | Fiber: 0 g | Cholesterol: 65 mg | Sodium: 210 mg | Phosphorus: 280 mg | Potassium: 420 mg.

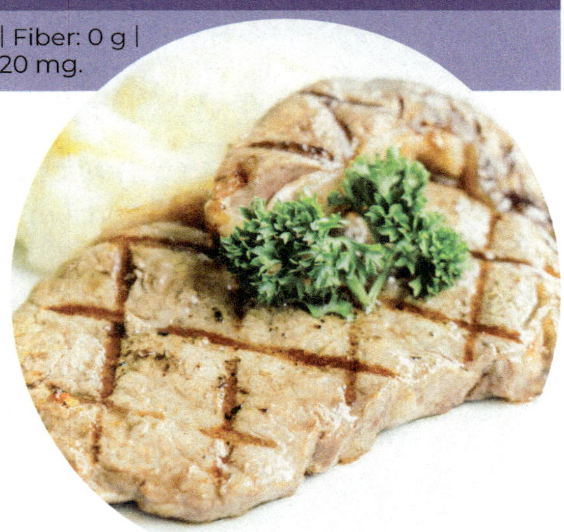

10 min | 14 min | 4

Ingredients:

- Four boneless pork chops (about 5 oz each)
- 2 tbsp Dijon mustard
- 1 tbsp olive oil
- 1 tbsp honey
- One garlic clove, minced
- Salt (ensure low sodium) and pepper to taste

Directions:

6. Preheat the grill or stovetop grill pan to medium-high heat.
7. Whisk together Dijon mustard, olive oil, honey, and minced garlic in a bowl.
8. Season each pork chop with salt and pepper, then brush the mustard glaze on both sides.
9. Grill the pork chops on each side for 6-7 minutes until they reach the desired doneness.
10. Serve immediately.

Heart-Healthy Benefits: *Pork is a fantastic source of critical vitamins and protein. Olive oil provides heart-healthy monounsaturated fats. Dijon mustard and honey offer flavor without the need for added sodium.*

NOTES

BEEF TENDERLOIN WITH ROASTED ASPARAGUS

Calories: 270 kCal | Protein: 31 g | Carbohydrates: 5 g | Sugar: 2 g | Fat: 15 g | Fiber: 2 g | Cholesterol: 85 mg | Sodium: 200 mg | Phosphorus: 310 mg | Potassium: 470 mg.

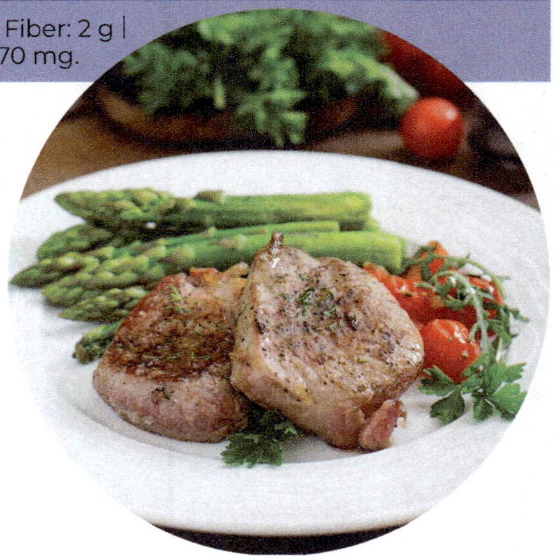

10 min | 25 min | 4

INGREDIENTS:

- 1 lb beef sirloin, cut into 1-inch cubes
- Three garlic cloves, minced
- 2 tbsp olive oil
- 1 tbsp fresh rosemary, finely chopped
- Salt (ensure low sodium) and pepper to taste

DIRECTIONS:

1. Preheat the oven to 400°F (205°C).
2. Toss the asparagus in 1 tbsp olive oil, lemon zest, salt, and pepper. Lay them on a baking sheet in a single layer.
3. Roast the asparagus in the oven for 15-20 minutes or until tender.
4. Over medium-high heat, warm the remaining olive oil in a skillet. Salt and pepper should be used to season the beef tenderloin steaks.
5. Cook the steaks on each side for 3-4 minutes or until desired doneness is achieved.
6. Serve steaks with roasted asparagus and a drizzle of fresh lemon juice.

Heart-Healthy Benefits: *Beef tenderloin is a lean cut, minimizing saturated fat intake. Vitamins, minerals, and antioxidants are abundant in asparagus. Olive oil and lemon provide heart-healthy fats and vitamin C, respectively.*

SAVORY HERB PORK RIBS (SLOW-COOKED)

Calories: 320 kCal | Protein: 24 g | Carbohydrates: 2 g | Sugar: 1 g | Fat: 24 g | Fiber: 0 g | Cholesterol: 90 mg | Sodium: 240 mg | Phosphorus: 260 mg | Potassium: 370 mg.

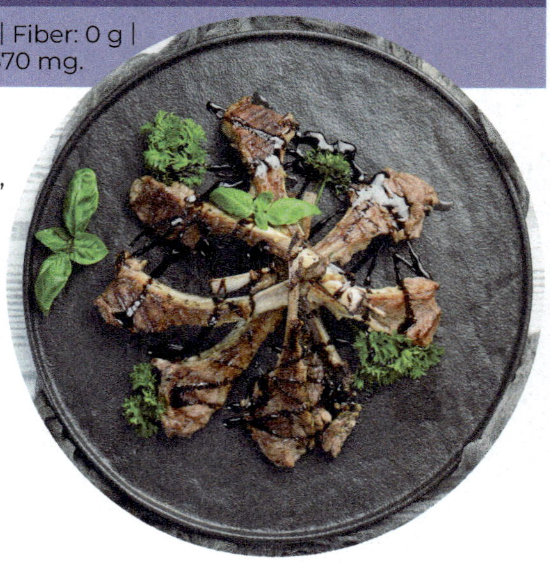

20 min | 4 hours (slow cooker) | 6

INGREDIENTS:

- 2 lbs pork ribs
- 2 tbsp olive oil
- 1 tbsp fresh rosemary, finely chopped
- 1 tbsp fresh thyme, finely chopped
- Three garlic cloves, minced
- Salt (ensure low sodium) and pepper to taste

DIRECTIONS:

7. In a mixing bowl, combine olive oil, rosemary, thyme, garlic, salt, and pepper.
8. Rub the herb mixture onto the ribs, ensuring all sides are coated.
9. Place the ribs in the slow cooker. Cover and cook on low for 4 hours or until tender.
10. Serve immediately.

Heart-Healthy Benefits: *Using a slow cooker reduces the need for additional fats. Fresh herbs like rosemary and thyme add antioxidants beneficial for heart health, and olive oil provides heart-healthy monounsaturated fats.*

NOTES

ASIAN INSPIRED BEEF & BROCCOLI

Calories: 260 kCal | Protein: 30 g | Carbohydrates: 10 g | Sugar: 4 g | Fat: 11 g | Fiber: 2 g | Cholesterol: 75 mg | Sodium: 180 mg | Phosphorus: 250 mg | Potassium: 480 mg.

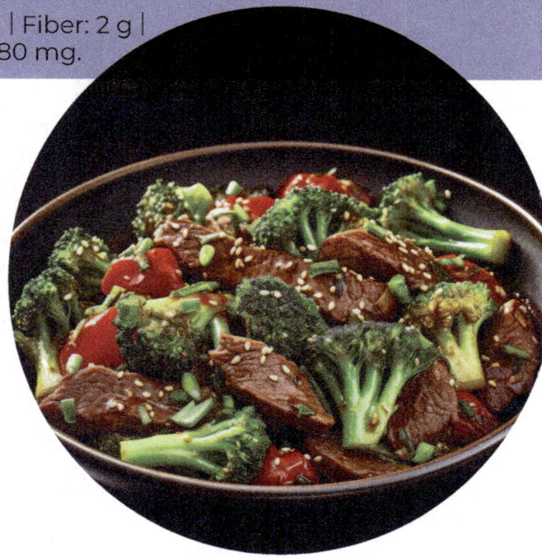

15 min | 12 min | 4

INGREDIENTS:

- 1 lb lean beef steak, thinly sliced
- 2 cups broccoli florets
- 3 tbsp low-sodium soy sauce
- 1 tbsp sesame oil
- Two garlic cloves, minced
- 1-inch fresh ginger, grated
- 1 tsp honey
- 1 tbsp sesame seeds
- Two green onions, thinly sliced

DIRECTIONS:

1. Mix soy sauce, sesame oil, minced garlic, grated ginger, and honey in a bowl.
2. Heat a wok or large skillet over medium-high heat. Add the beef slices and stir-fry until nearly cooked, about 2-3 minutes.
3. Add the broccoli florets to the pan and pour the sauce mixture over. Stir-fry until the beef is fully cooked and broccoli is tender-crisp, about 4-5 minutes.
4. Before serving, add sliced green onions and sesame seeds as a garnish.

Heart-Healthy Benefits: *Lean beef cuts reduce saturated fat intake, while broccoli provides a host of vitamins and antioxidants beneficial for heart health. Soy sauce adds flavor without additional salt, and ginger contains anti-inflammatory properties.*

BEEF SIRLOIN & CARAMELIZED ONION BITES

Calories: 190 kCal | Protein: 20 g | Carbohydrates: 8 g | Sugar: 5 g | Fat: 8 g | Fiber: 1 g | Cholesterol: 50 mg | Sodium: 100 mg | Phosphorus: 210 mg | Potassium: 310 mg.

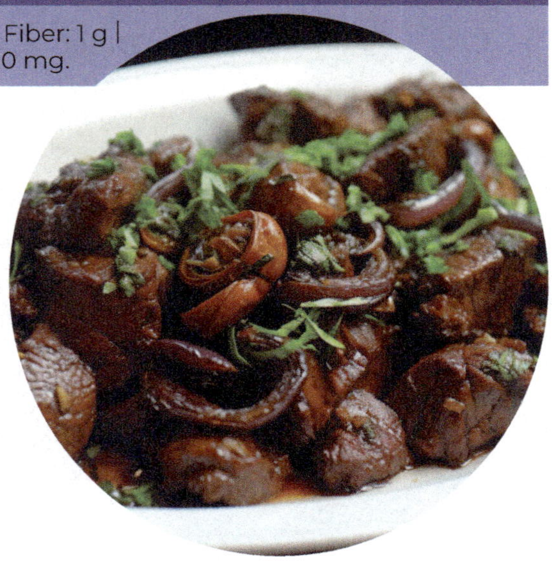

10 min | 20 min | 6

INGREDIENTS:

- 1 lb beef sirloin, cut into bite-sized pieces
- Two large onions, thinly sliced
- 1 tbsp olive oil
- 1/4 cup balsamic vinegar
- Salt (ensure low sodium) and freshly ground black pepper to taste
- Fresh thyme for garnish

DIRECTIONS:

5. Olive oil is heated in a skillet at a medium temperature. Sliced onions should be added and cooked until they start to soften.
6. The onions should be caramelized and deeply browned before adding balsamic vinegar and continuing to cook. Stirring occasionally is recommended.
7. Season beef sirloin bites with salt and pepper. Push the onions to one side of the skillet and add the beef. Cook until browned on all sides.
8. Serve beef and caramelized onion bites garnished with fresh thyme.

Heart-Healthy Benefits: *Beef sirloin is a lean cut that provides essential proteins and amino acids. Onions are rich in antioxidants and have been linked to heart health benefits, particularly when caramelized with balsamic vinegar, which adds a sweet depth and contains polyphenols known for their heart-friendly properties.*

CUMIN LIME PORK STEAKS

Calories: 260 kCal | Protein: 25 g | Carbohydrates: 3 g | Sugar: 1 g | Fat: 17 g | Fiber: 0 g | Cholesterol: 75 mg | Sodium: 90 mg | Phosphorus: 220 mg | Potassium: 360 mg.

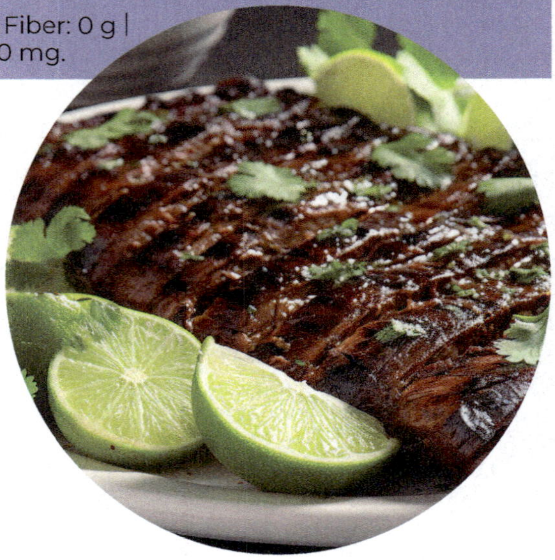

15 min (plus marination) | 10 min | 4

INGREDIENTS:

- 1 lb pork steaks
- Juice of 2 limes
- 2 tsp cumin powder
- Three garlic cloves, minced
- 2 tbsp olive oil
- Salt (ensure low sodium) and freshly ground black pepper to taste
- Fresh cilantro leaves for garnish

DIRECTIONS:

1. Whisk together lime juice, cumin, minced garlic, olive oil, salt, and pepper to form a marinade.
2. Place the pork steaks in the marinade, ensuring each piece is well-coated. Cover and refrigerate for at least 1 hour.
3. Preheat a grill or skillet over medium-high heat. Cook the pork steaks on each side for 4-5 minutes until they reach the desired doneness.
4. Serve the steaks hot, garnished with fresh cilantro leaves.

Heart-Healthy Benefits: *B vitamins and essential minerals like potassium and phosphorus are abundant in pork. Cumin is known to have anti-inflammatory properties, and lime provides a burst of vitamin C. Together, these ingredients promote a heart-healthy meal.*

SOY-GINGER GLAZED PORK SKEWERS

Calories: 225 kCal | Protein: 26 g | Carbohydrates: 7 g | Sugar: 5 g | Fat: 9 g | Fiber: 1 g | Cholesterol: 70 mg | Sodium: 350 mg | Phosphorus: 280 mg | Potassium: 370 mg.

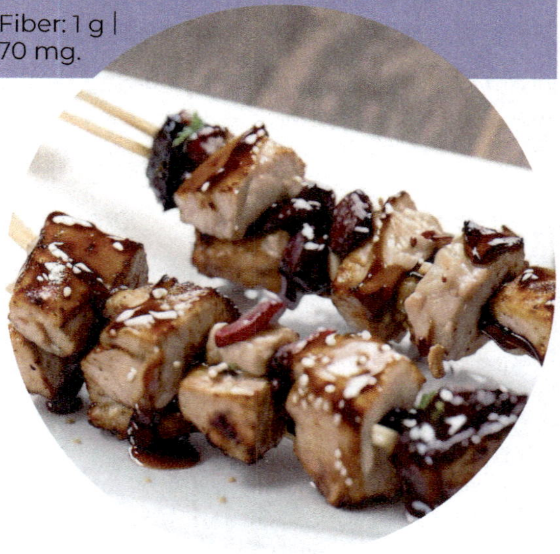

20 min (plus marination) | 12 min | 4

INGREDIENTS:

- 1 lb pork loin, cut into 1-inch cubes
- 3 tbsp low-sodium soy sauce
- 2 tbsp fresh ginger, grated
- Two garlic cloves, minced
- 1 tbsp honey
- Two green onions, finely chopped
- 1 tbsp sesame oil

DIRECTIONS:

1. Mix low-sodium soy sauce, grated ginger, minced garlic, honey, green onions, and sesame oil in a bowl.
2. Add the pork cubes to the mixture, ensuring they are well-coated. Cover and marinate in the refrigerator for at least 2 hours.
3. Preheat grill or broiler. Thread the pork cubes onto skewers.
4. Grill or broil the skewers for 6 minutes on each side or until fully cooked, occasionally basting with any remaining marinade.
5. Serve hot with steamed veggies or a side salad.

Heart-Healthy Benefits: *Pork loin is a lean protein source for muscle health and overall body maintenance. Ginger and garlic offer anti-inflammatory properties, which can aid heart health. The use of low-sodium soy sauce ensures a flavorful yet sodium-conscious dish.*

NOTES

BEEF & BELL PEPPER KEBABS

Calories: 290 kCal | Protein: 27 g | Carbohydrates: 5 g | Sugar: 3 g | Fat: 18 g | Fiber: 1 g | Cholesterol: 70 mg | Sodium: 90 mg | Phosphorus: 230 mg | Potassium: 350 mg.

20 min | 10 min | 4

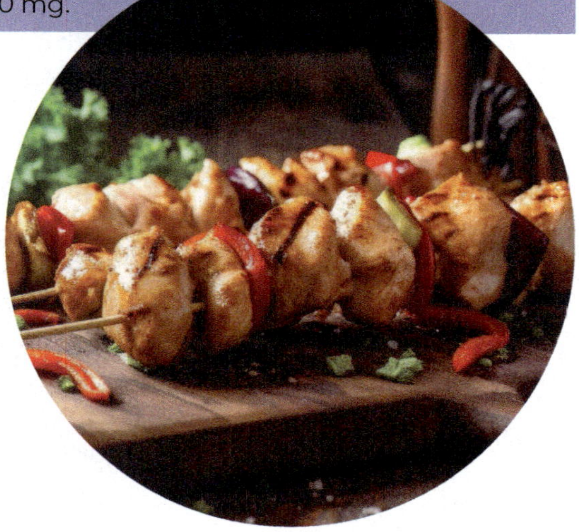

INGREDIENTS:

- 1 lb beef sirloin, cut into 1-inch cubes
- Two bell peppers (any color), cut into 1-inch pieces
- 1/4 cup olive oil
- 2 tbsp lemon juice
- 1 tsp dried oregano
- Salt (ensure low sodium) and freshly ground black pepper to taste

DIRECTIONS:

1. Whisk together olive oil, lemon juice, oregano, salt, and pepper in a bowl.
2. Add beef cubes to the marinade, ensuring they are well-coated. Let them marinate for at least 1 hour.
3. Preheat grill or broiler. Alternate threading beef cubes and bell pepper pieces onto skewers.
4. Grill or broil the kebabs on each side for 4-5 minutes or until the beef is cooked to the desired level.
5. Serve immediately with a side of quinoa or whole-grain rice.

Heart-Healthy Benefits: *Beef sirloin offers lean protein and essential amino acids. Vitamin C, an antioxidant that aids in heart protection, is abundant in bell peppers. Olive oil provides heart-healthy monounsaturated fats that can help to reduce harmful cholesterol levels.*

BEEF & MUSHROOM STUFFED TOMATOES

Calories: 180 kCal | Protein: 20 g | Carbohydrates: 10 g | Sugar: 5 g | Fat: 7 g | Fiber: 2 g | Cholesterol: 50 mg | Sodium: 90 mg | Phosphorus: 250 mg | Potassium: 600 mg.

20 min | 25 min | 4

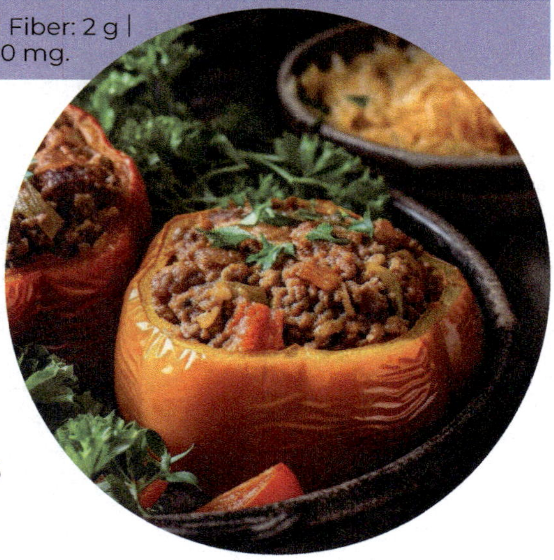

INGREDIENTS:

- Four large tomatoes
- 1/2 lb lean ground beef
- 1 cup mushrooms, finely chopped
- One small onion, finely chopped
- Two garlic cloves, minced
- 1 tbsp olive oil
- Fresh basil for garnish
- Salt (ensure low sodium) and freshly ground black pepper to taste

DIRECTIONS:

1. Preheat the oven to 375°F (190°C).
2. Slice off the top of each tomato and gently scoop out the inside, leaving a shell. Set aside.
3. Olive oil is heated in a skillet at a medium temperature. Add onions and garlic and sauté until translucent.
4. Brown the ground beef after adding it. Add the mushrooms and continue to cook for another 5 minutes.
5. Season the beef and mushroom mixture with minimal salt and pepper.
6. Fill each tomato shell with the beef and mushroom mixture and place them in a baking dish.
7. Bake in the oven for 20-25 minutes or until the tomatoes are tender.
8. Garnish with fresh basil and serve.

Heart-Healthy Benefits: *Lycopene, an antioxidant that helps to improve heart health, is found in tomatoes in significant amounts. Mushrooms offer beneficial nutrients like selenium and potassium, which are heart-friendly. Olive oil contains monounsaturated fats that can help lower harmful cholesterol levels.*

Seafood Recipes

HERB-STEAMED MUSSELS WITH LEMON ZEST

Calories: 210 kCal | Protein: 22 g | Carbohydrates: 6 g | Sugar: 1 g | Fat: 4 g | Fiber: 0,2 g | Cholesterol: 50 mg | Sodium: 400 mg | Phosphorus: 280 mg | Potassium: 500 mg.

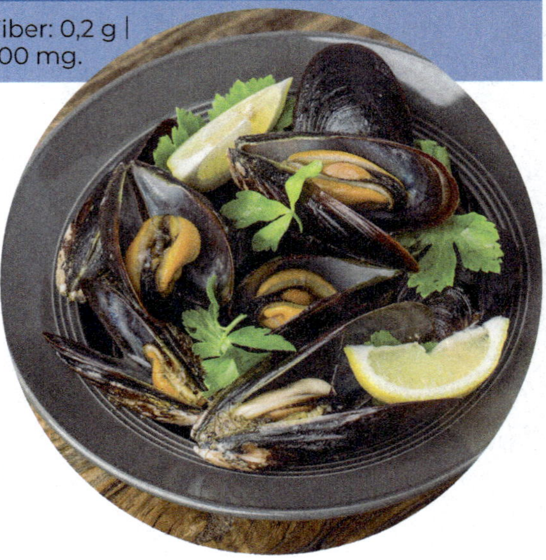

15 min | 10 min | 4

Ingredients:

- 2 pounds fresh mussels, cleaned and de-bearded
- 1 cup white wine (choose a good quality dry white like Sauvignon Blanc)
- Two garlic cloves, minced
- 1/4 cup fresh parsley, chopped
- Zest of 1 lemon
- One tablespoon of olive oil
- Freshly ground black pepper
- A pinch of sea salt (optional)

Directions:

1. In a large pot, heat olive oil over medium heat. Add garlic and sauté until fragrant.
2. Add white wine, lemon zest, and mussels to the pot. Cover and let steam until mussels have opened, about 6-8 minutes.
3. Discard any mussels that haven't opened.
4. Transfer mussels to serving plates and sprinkle with fresh parsley and ground black pepper.
5. If desired, you can drizzle a bit of the wine broth over the mussels.

Heart-Healthy Benefits: *Mussels have high omega-3 fatty acids, which are believed to lower the risk of heart disease. Garlic has been linked to reduced cholesterol and blood pressure. White wine, in moderation, contains antioxidants beneficial for heart health. Parsley and lemon provide vitamin C and other antioxidants.*

CILANTRO-LIME GRILLED PRAWNS

Calories: 210 kCal | Protein: 22 g | Carbohydrates: 6 g | Sugar: 1 g | Fat: 4 g | Fiber: 0,2 g | Cholesterol: 50 mg | Sodium: 400 mg | Phosphorus: 280 mg | Potassium: 500 mg.

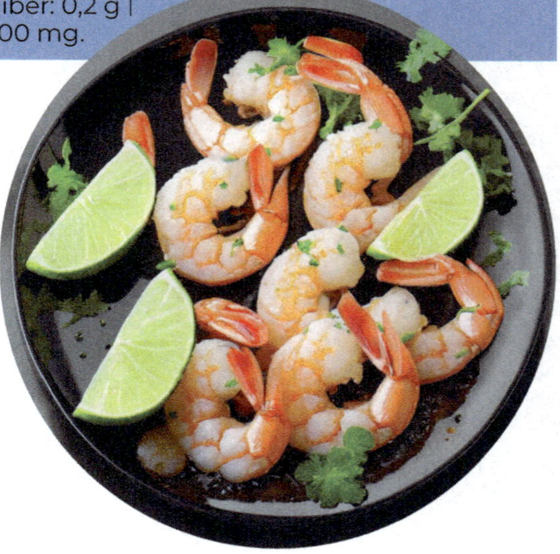

20 min (plus marination) | 5 min | 4

Ingredients:

- 1.5 pounds large prawns, peeled and deveined
- 1/4 cup fresh cilantro, finely chopped
- Zest and juice of 2 limes
- Two tablespoons of olive oil
- Two garlic cloves, minced
- A pinch of sea salt and black pepper

Directions:

1. Combine cilantro, zest, lime juice, olive oil, garlic, salt, and pepper in a mixing bowl. Mix well.
2. Add prawns to the bowl and toss until they're well-coated. Let marinate for at least 30 minutes.
3. Preheat the grill to medium-high heat. Grill prawns on each side for 2-3 minutes until they turn pink and are opaque.
4. Serve immediately, garnished with additional cilantro and lime wedges.

Heart-Healthy Benefits: *Prawns are a lean source of protein, which is beneficial for heart health.*

SHRIMP & AVOCADO LETTUCE WRAPS

Calories: 250 kCal | Protein: 20 g | Carbohydrates: 12 g | Sugar: 3 g | Fat: 16 g | Fiber: 7 g | Cholesterol: 145 mg | Sodium: 180 mg | Phosphorus: 190 mg | Potassium: 500 mg.

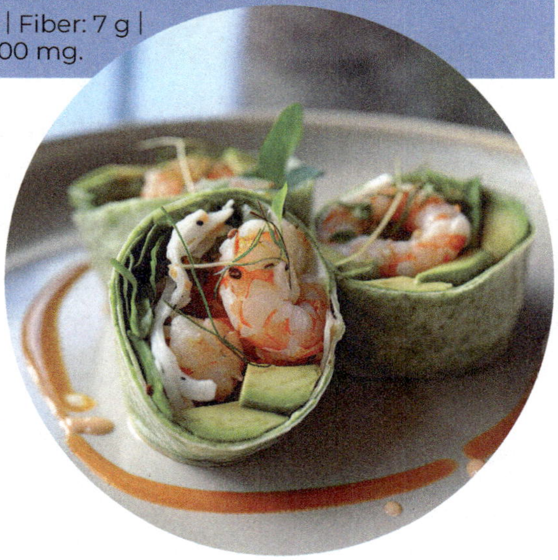

20 min | 5 min | 4

INGREDIENTS:

- 1 pound large shrimp, peeled and deveined
- Two ripe avocados, diced
- One red bell pepper, diced
- 1/4 cup fresh cilantro, chopped
- Juice of 2 limes
- One tablespoon of olive oil
- One clove of garlic, minced
- One head of butter lettuce
- Freshly ground black pepper and a pinch of sea salt

DIRECTIONS:

1. In a pan, heat olive oil over medium heat. Add garlic and sauté until fragrant. Add shrimp and cook for 2-3 minutes on each side or until they turn pink. Remove from heat.
2. Combine avocado, bell pepper, cilantro, and lime juice in a mixing bowl. Season with salt and pepper.
3. Carefully peel the leaves from the lettuce head to create "cups."
4. To assemble, place a few shrimps into each lettuce cup and top with avocado mixture.
5. Serve immediately with a wedge of lime on the side.

Heart-Healthy Benefits: *Omega-3 fatty acids, which are suitable for the heart, are found in shrimp, a lean source of protein. Avocados are a good source of potassium and monounsaturated fats, which are ideal for the soul. The antioxidants found in bell peppers and cilantro also promote cardiovascular well-being.*

GARLIC BUTTER LOBSTER TAILS

Note: While traditional garlic butter is off-limits due to butter restrictions, we'll use a heart-healthy olive oil alternative.

Calories: 210 kCal | Protein: 24 g | Carbohydrates: 1 g | Sugar: 0 g | Fat: 12 g | Fiber: 0,1 g | Cholesterol: 80 mg | Sodium: 220 mg | Phosphorus: 250 mg | Potassium: 380 mg.

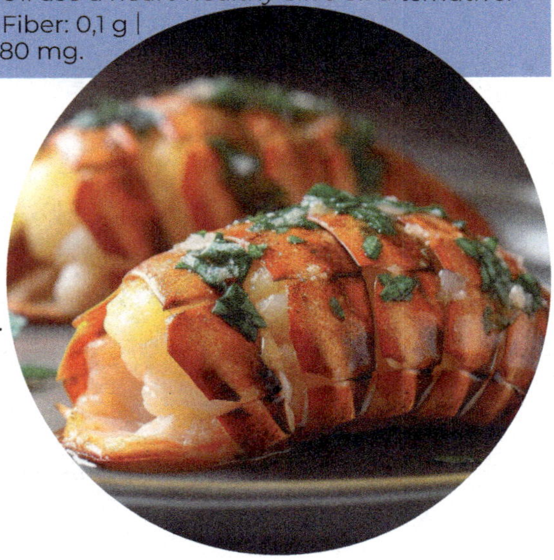

15 min | 15 min | 4

INGREDIENTS:

- Four lobster tails split lengthwise
- 1/4 cup olive oil
- Three garlic cloves, minced
- 1/4 cup fresh parsley, finely chopped
- Zest and juice of 1 lemon
- Freshly ground black pepper and a pinch of sea salt

DIRECTIONS:

1. Preheat your grill to medium-high heat.
2. Whisk together olive oil, garlic, parsley, lemon zest, and lemon juice in a bowl. Season with a touch of sea salt and black pepper.
3. Brush the lobster tails with the olive oil, ensuring some in the flesh.
4. Place the lobster tails, flesh side down, on the grill. Grill for 5-7 minutes. Flip, brush again with the garlic mixture, and grill for 5-7 minutes or until the meat is opaque.
5. Serve immediately with a squeeze of lemon and some chopped fresh parsley.

Heart-Healthy Benefits: *Lobster is a lean protein source and contains vital minerals, including selenium, which is beneficial for heart health. Olive oil offers heart-healthy monounsaturated fats and antioxidants.*

MEDITERRANEAN SHRIMP & VEGETABLE SKEWERS

Calories: 230 kCal | Protein: 25 g | Carbohydrates: 10 g | Sugar: 5 g | Fat: 11 g | Fiber: 2 g | Cholesterol: 170 mg | Sodium: 200 mg | Phosphorus: 290 mg | Potassium: 460 mg.

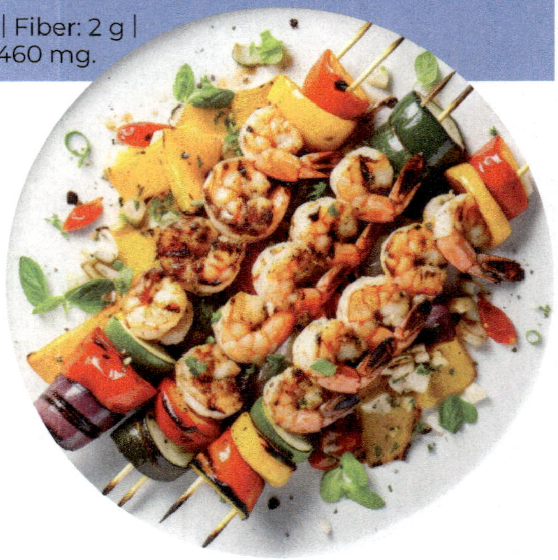

20 min | 10 min | 4

INGREDIENTS:

- 1 pound large shrimp, peeled and deveined
- One zucchini cut into 1-inch rounds
- One red bell pepper cut into 1-inch squares
- One yellow bell pepper cut into 1-inch squares
- One red onion, cut into wedges
- 1/4 cup olive oil
- Two garlic cloves, minced
- Two teaspoons of dried oregano
- Zest and juice of 1 lemon
- Sea salt and freshly ground black pepper

DIRECTIONS:

1. Combine olive oil, garlic, oregano, lemon zest, and lemon juice in a bowl. Season with a touch of sea salt and black pepper.
2. Thread the shrimp, zucchini, bell peppers, and onion alternately onto skewers. Brush the skewers with the olive oil mixture.
3. Preheat the grill to medium-high heat. Place skewers on the grill, cooking for 2-3 minutes per side or until shrimp turns pink and vegetables are slightly charred.
4. Serve immediately with quinoa or a crisp green salad.

Heart-Healthy Benefits: *Shrimp is rich in omega-3 fatty acids, which can improve heart health. The colorful bell peppers and zucchini provide essential vitamins, antioxidants, and fiber that support cardiovascular health. Olive oil contains heart-friendly monounsaturated fats.*

BASIL & TOMATO SHRIMP BRUSCHETTA

Calories: 240 kCal | Protein: 25 g | Carbohydrates: 20 g | Sugar: 3 g | Fat: 8 g | Fiber: 3 g | Cholesterol: 170 mg | Sodium: 200 mg | Phosphorus: 240 mg | Potassium: 370 mg.

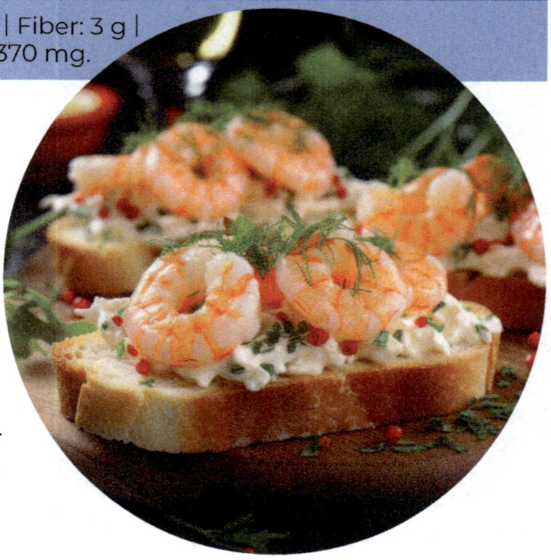

20 min | 5 min | 4

INGREDIENTS:

- 1 pound large shrimp, peeled and deveined
- Two medium tomatoes, diced
- 1/4 cup fresh basil, chopped
- Two tablespoons of olive oil
- Two garlic cloves, minced
- One tablespoon of balsamic vinegar
- 1/4 teaspoon sea salt
- 1/4 teaspoon freshly ground black pepper
- Four slices of whole-grain bread

DIRECTIONS:

5. Preheat a grill or skillet to medium-high heat.
6. Combine the tomatoes, basil, garlic, balsamic vinegar, salt, pepper, and one tablespoon of olive oil in a bowl. Mix well and set aside.
7. Add the remaining tablespoon of olive oil to the shrimp and toss before cooking them on the grill or in a skillet. Cook for 2-3 minutes on each side until they turn pink.
8. Toast the whole-grain bread slices until they are crispy.
9. Top each slice of bread with a generous spoonful of the tomato-basil mixture. Place grilled shrimp on top and serve immediately.

Heart-Healthy Benefits: *When consumed in moderation, shrimp can be a heart-healthy protein source. Tomatoes provide lycopene, an antioxidant linked to heart health, while basil and whole-grain bread offer dietary fiber essential for cardiovascular well-being.*

LEMON HERB BAKED SALMON

Calories: 280 kCal | Protein: 34 g | Carbohydrates: 2 g | Sugar: 1 g | Fat: 16 g | Fiber: 0 g | Cholesterol: 70 mg | Sodium: 160 mg | Phosphorus: 50 mg | Potassium: 570 mg.

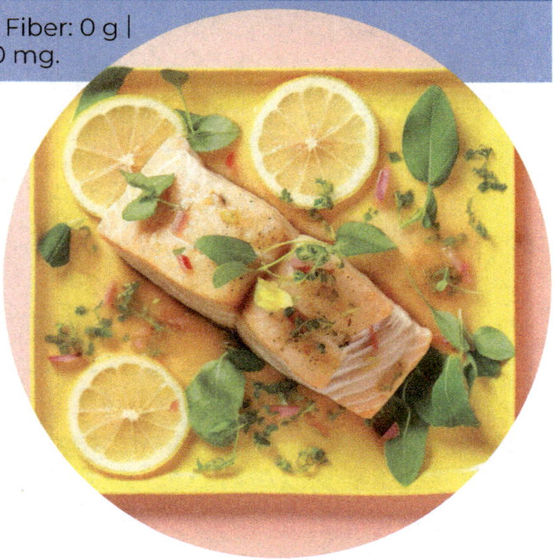

10 min | 20 min | 4

Ingredients:

- Four salmon fillets
- 2 tbsp olive oil
- Zest and juice of 1 lemon
- Two garlic cloves, minced
- 1 tbsp chopped fresh dill
- 1 tbsp chopped fresh parsley
- Salt to taste (keep sodium below 20% per serving)

Directions:

1. Preheat the oven to 400°F (205°C).
2. Mix olive oil, lemon zest, lemon juice, garlic, dill, parsley, and salt in a small bowl.
3. In a baking dish, put the salmon fillets and the herb mixture.
4. Bke in the oven for 20 minutes or until salmon flakes easily with a fork.

Heart-Healthy Benefits: *Omega-3 fatty acids, which can lower blood pressure, reduce inflammation, and cut the risk of heart disease, are a great source of nutrition in salmon.*

HONEY-GINGER GLAZED TILAPIA

Calories: 210 kCal | Protein: 28 g | Carbohydrates: 10 g | Sugar: 8 g | Fat: 6 g | Fiber: 0 g | Cholesterol: 60 mg | Sodium: 190 mg | Phosphorus: 40 mg | Potassium: 380 mg.

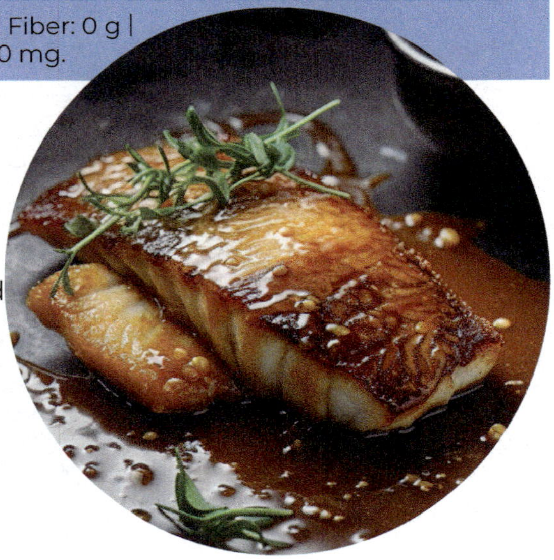

15 min | 15 min | 4

Ingredients:

- Four tilapia fillets
- 2 tbsp honey
- 1-inch ginger, grated
- 2 tbsp low-sodium soy sauce
- 1 tbsp olive oil
- Two green onions, sliced

Directions:

1. In a bowl, mix honey, ginger, and soy sauce.
2. Heat olive oil in a skillet over medium heat.
3. Place tilapia fillets in the skillet and cook for 3 minutes on each side.
4. Pour the honey-ginger mixture over the tilapia and cook for another 2 minutes until the fish is glazed and cooked.
5. Serve topped with sliced green onions.

Heart-Healthy Benefits: *Tilapia is a lean protein source, and ginger offers anti-inflammatory properties that can promote heart health.*

NOTES

BALSAMIC GLAZED RAINBOW TROUT

Calories: 230 kCal | Protein: 31 g | Carbohydrates: 3 g | Sugar: 2 g | Fat: 11 g | Fiber: 0 g | Cholesterol: 70 mg | Sodium: 150 mg | Phosphorus: 50 mg | Potassium: 510 mg.

10 min | 15 min | 4

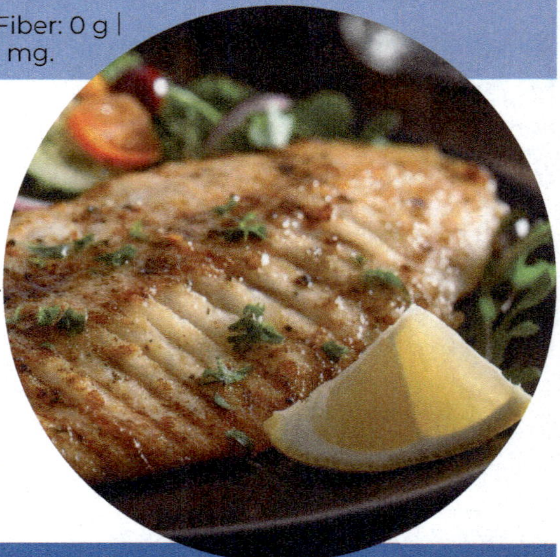

INGREDIENTS:

- Two rainbow trout fillets
- 2 tbsp balsamic vinegar
- 1 tbsp olive oil
- One garlic clove, minced
- Salt to taste (keep sodium below 20% per serving)

DIRECTIONS:

1. Heat olive oil in a skillet over medium heat.
2. Add trout fillets skin-side down and cook for 3 minutes.
3. Flip the fillets and cook for another 2 minutes.
4. Pour balsamic vinegar and add garlic to the skillet. Cook for 2-3 minutes until trout is glazed.

Heart-Healthy Benefits: *Rainbow trout is another excellent source of omega-3 fatty acids for heart health.*

ZESTY ORANGE BAKED MACKEREL

Calories: 240 kCal | Protein: 22 g | Carbohydrates: 4 g | Sugar: 3 g | Fat: 15 g | Fiber: 0 g | Cholesterol: 70 mg | Sodium: 180 mg | Phosphorus: 60 mg | Potassium: 520 mg.

20 min | 5 min | 4

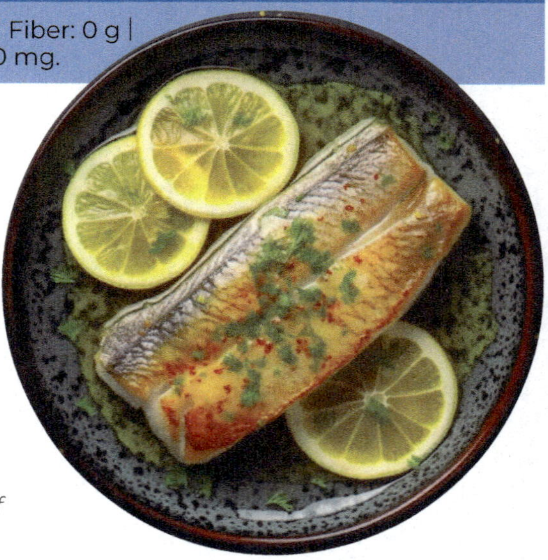

INGREDIENTS:

- Four mackerel fillets
- Zest and juice of 1 orange
- 2 tbsp olive oil
- 1 tsp paprika
- Salt to taste (keep sodium below 20% per serving)

DIRECTIONS:

1. Preheat the oven to 375°F (190°C).
2. Whisk together the orange zest, orange juice, olive oil, paprika, and salt in a bowl.
3. Place mackerel fillets in a baking dish and pour the orange mixture over them.
4. Bake for 20 minutes or until the mackerel is cooked through.

Heart-Healthy Benefits: *Mackerel is one of the wealthiest providers of omega-3 fatty acids, which are known to be good for the heart.*

TUSCAN HERB GRILLED SARDINES

Calories: 210 kCal | Protein: 24 g | Carbohydrates: 1 g | Sugar: 0 g | Fat: 13 g | Fiber: 0 g | Cholesterol: 50 mg | Sodium: 160 mg | Phosphorus: 40 mg | Potassium: 490 mg.

10 min | 10 min | 4

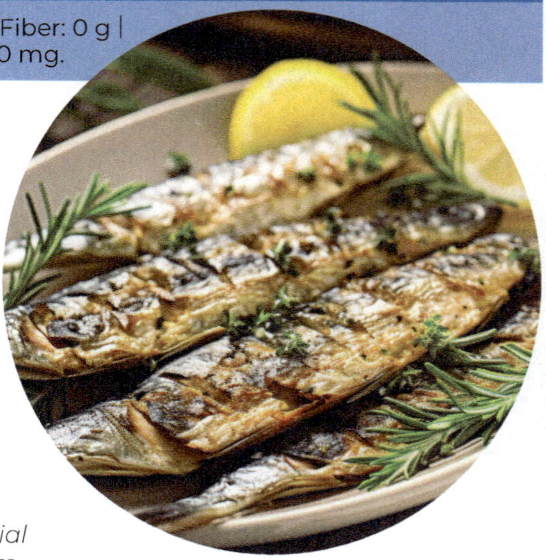

INGREDIENTS:

- Six whole sardines, cleaned
- 1 tbsp olive oil
- 1 tsp chopped rosemary
- 1 tsp chopped thyme
- 1 tsp chopped oregano
- Salt to taste (keep sodium below 20% per serving)

DIRECTIONS:

1. Preheat the grill to medium-high heat.
2. Mix olive oil, rosemary, thyme, oregano, and salt in a bowl.
3. Brush sardines with the herb mixture.
4. Place sardines on the grill and cook for 5 minutes on each side.

Heart-Healthy Benefits: *Sardines are rich in various nutrients beneficial for the heart, including omega-3 fatty acids, vitamin B12, and selenium.*

THYME & LEMON GRILLED GROUPER

Calories: 230 kCal | Protein: 30 g | Carbohydrates: 2 g | Sugar: 1 g | Fat: 11 g | Fiber: 0 g | Cholesterol: 60 mg | Sodium: 170 mg | Phosphorus: 55 mg | Potassium: 540 mg.

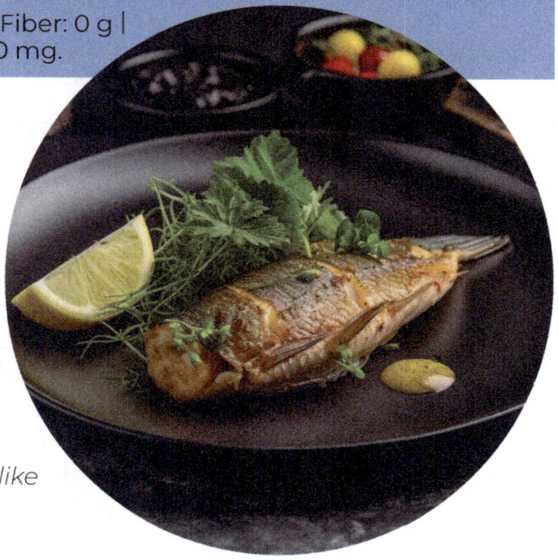

15 min | 15 min | 4

Ingredients:

- Four grouper fillets
- 2 tbsp olive oil
- Zest and juice of 1 lemon
- 1 tbsp fresh thyme leaves
- Salt to taste (keep sodium below 20% per serving)

Directions:

1. Preheat the grill to medium-high heat.
2. In a bowl, combine olive oil, lemon zest, lemon juice, thyme, and salt.
3. Rub the mixture onto the grouper fillets.
4. Grill for 7 minutes on each side or until the fish is cooked.

Heart-Healthy Benefits: *People who consume lean protein from fish like grouper are less likely to gain weight and develop heart disease.*

ROSEMARY INFUSED BAKED POLLOCK

Calories: 220 kCal | Protein: 26 g | Carbohydrates: 1 g | Sugar: 0 g | Fat: 12 g | Fiber: 0 g | Cholesterol: 65 mg | Sodium: 180 mg | Phosphorus: 50 mg | Potassium: 480 mg.

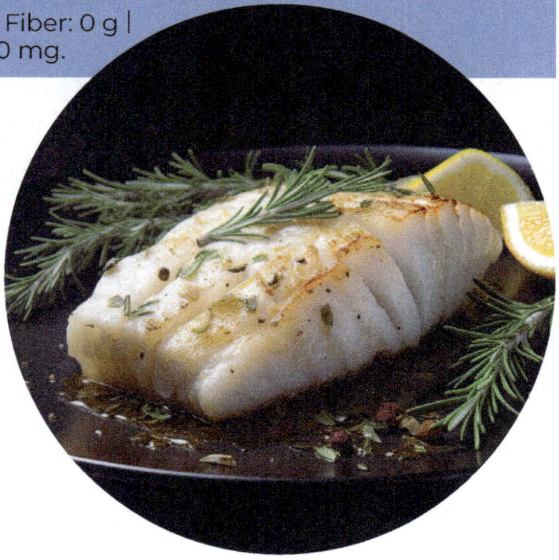

10 min | 20 min | 4

Ingredients:

- Four pollock fillets
- 2 tbsp olive oil
- Two sprigs of fresh rosemary, finely chopped
- One clove of garlic, minced
- Salt to taste (keep sodium below 20% per serving)
- Zest of 1 lemon

Directions:

1. Preheat the oven to 375°F (190°C).
2. Mix olive oil, rosemary, garlic, and lemon zest in a bowl.
3. Place the pollock fillets in a baking dish and drizzle with the rosemary mixture.
4. Bake for 20 minutes or until the pollock is flaky and cooked through.

Heart-Healthy Benefits: *Pollock, a white fish, is a good source of lean protein and B vitamins. Rosemary is packed with antioxidants that have potential heart-protective properties.*

NOTES

LEMON BUTTER SEARED SALMON FILLETS

Calories: 290 kCal | Protein: 25 g | Carbohydrates: 2 g | Sugar: 1 g | Fat: 20 g | Fiber: 0,5 g | Cholesterol: 75 mg | Sodium: 50 mg | Phosphorus: 370 mg | Potassium: 650 mg.

15 min | 10 min | 4

INGREDIENTS:

- Four salmon fillets
- Two tablespoons of olive oil
- Juice and zest of 1 lemon
- One tablespoon of fresh dill, chopped
- Black pepper to taste

DIRECTIONS:

1. Combine olive oil, lemon juice, lemon zest, dill, and black pepper in a bowl.
2. Marinate the salmon fillets in this mixture for 10 minutes.
3. Preheat a non-stick skillet over medium heat.
4. Remove salmon from the marinade and place in the skillet.
5. Sear for 4-5 minutes on each side or until golden and cooked to your preference.
6. Serve immediately.

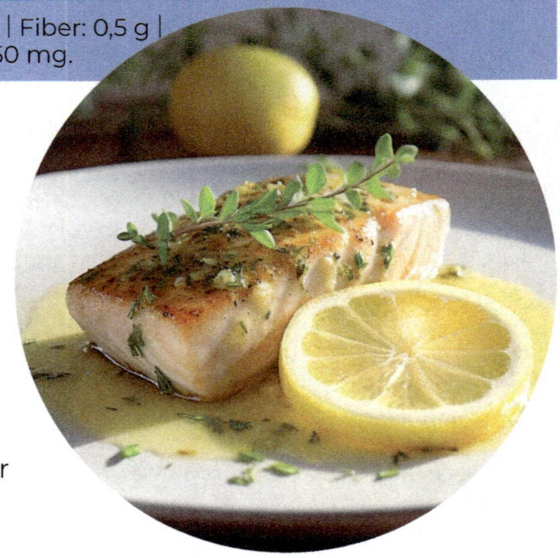

Heart-Healthy Benefits: *Salmon is renowned for its dense concentration of omega-3 fatty acids. These help decrease inflammation, lower blood pressure, and reduce the risk of clotting — pivotal in maintaining good heart health. Dill and lemon provide zesty flavor without the need for excessive salt.*

CUMIN & LIME BAKED CATFISH

Calories: 190 kCal | Protein: 20 g | Carbohydrates: 1 g | Sugar: 0 g | Fat: 11 g | Fiber: 0 g | Cholesterol: 60 mg | Sodium: 50 mg | Phosphorus: 340 mg | Potassium: 450 mg.

10 min | 20 min | 4

INGREDIENTS:

- Four catfish fillets
- One tablespoon of olive oil
- Juice and zest of 1 lime
- One teaspoon of ground cumin
- 1/2 teaspoon black pepper
- Fresh cilantro, chopped for garnish

DIRECTIONS:

1. Preheat oven to 375°F (190°C).
2. Mix olive oil, lime juice, lime zest, cumin, and black pepper in a bowl.
3. Arrange catfish fillets in a baking dish and pour the mixture over them.
4. Bake in the oven for 20 minutes or until the fish is flaky.
5. Garnish with fresh cilantro before serving.

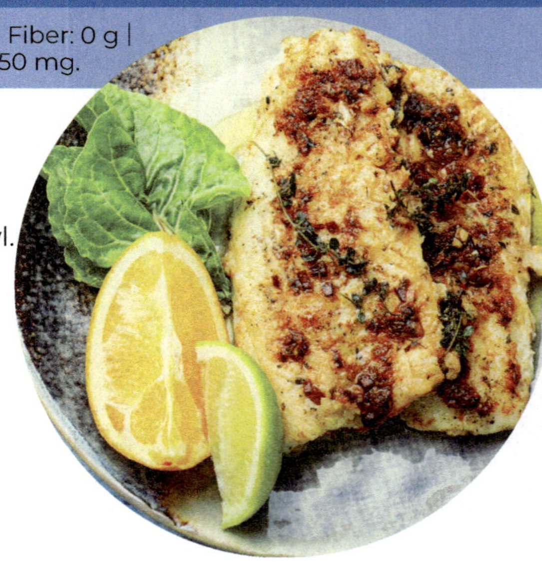

Heart-Healthy Benefits: *Catfish provides a lean source of protein. The addition of cumin not only adds flavor but may have anti-inflammatory properties. Lime provides a tangy flavor, which negates the need for additional salt.*

NOTES

HERBAL BERRY INFUSION

Calories: 10 kCal | Protein: 0 g | Carbohydrates: 2 g | Sugar: 1 g | Fat: 0 g | Fiber: 0,5 g | Cholesterol: 0 mg | Sodium: 10 mg | Phosphorus: 5 mg | Potassium: 15 mg.

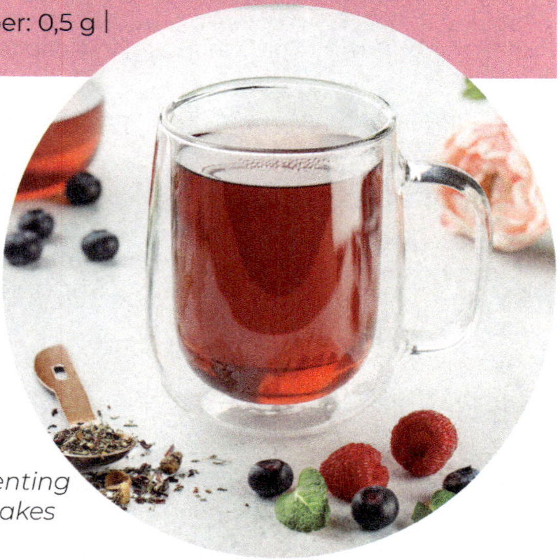

5 min | 5 min | 4
(Steep time: 10 min)

INGREDIENTS:

- 1-quart boiling water
- Two herbal berry tea bags (like a blend of hibiscus, rosehips, and berries)
- Fresh mixed berries (raspberries, blueberries, strawberries) for garnish

DIRECTIONS:

1. Pour boiling water into a teapot or pitcher over the tea bags.
2. Allow to steep for 10 minutes.
3. Remove tea bags and let the infusion cool.
4. Serve in glasses, garnished with fresh mixed berries.

Heart-Healthy Benefits: *Berry infusions are rich in antioxidants, preventing chronic diseases and defending the heart. The absence of caffeine makes this an excellent choice for those looking to manage blood pressure.*

GREEN TEA & GINGER COOLER

Calories: 10 kCal | Protein: 0 g | Carbohydrates: 3 g | Sugar: 0 g | Fat: 13 g | Fiber: 0,5 g | Cholesterol: 0 mg | Sodium: 10 mg | Phosphorus: 5 mg | Potassium: 40 mg.

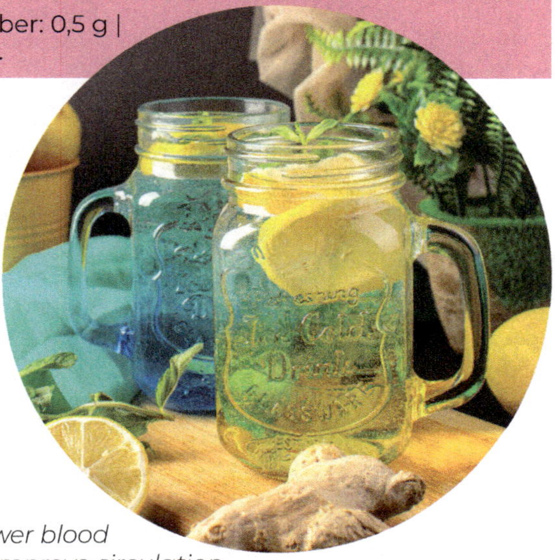

5 min | 5 min | 4
(chill time: 2 hours)

INGREDIENTS:

- Four green tea bags
- 1 gallon filtered water
- 2-inch piece of fresh ginger, thinly sliced
- One lemon, thinly sliced

DIRECTIONS:

1. Boil the filtered water in a pot.
2. Once boiling, remove from heat and add the green tea bags and ginger slices. Allow to steep for about 5 minutes.
3. Remove the tea bags and let the tea cool down to room temperature.
4. Transfer the tea to a pitcher, add lemon slices, and refrigerate for at least 2 hours.
5. Serve chilled.

Heart-Healthy Benefits: *Green tea has many catechins, which help lower blood pressure and cholesterol. The anti-inflammatory effects of ginger can improve circulation.*

REFRESHING CUCUMBER MINT WATER

Calories: 5 kCal | Protein: 0 g | Carbohydrates: 1 g | Sugar: 0 g | Fat: 0 g | Fiber: 0 g | Cholesterol: 0 mg | Sodium: 5 mg | Phosphorus: 10 mg | Potassium: 40 mg.

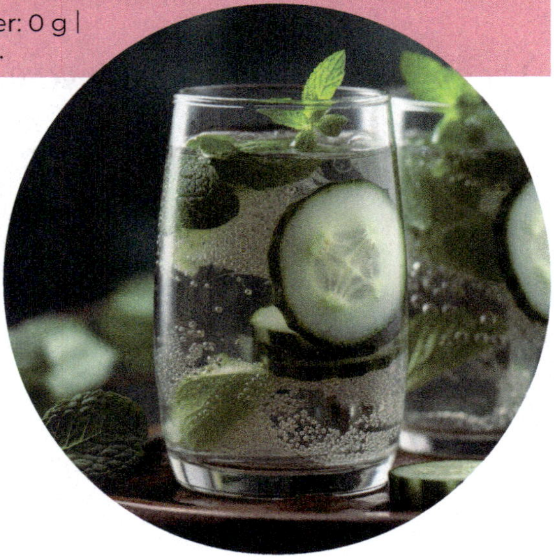

5 min | 0 min | 4
(chill time: 2 hours)

INGREDIENTS:

- One cucumber, thinly sliced
- Ten fresh mint leaves
- 1 gallon filtered water

DIRECTIONS:

1. Pour boiling water into a teapot or pitcher over the tea bags.
2. Allow to steep for 10 minutes.
3. Remove tea bags and let the infusion cool.
4. Serve in glasses, garnished with fresh mixed berries.

Heart-Healthy Benefits: *Cucumbers and mint are hydrating and help reduce bloating. The absence of sugar and the natural infusion make this a heart-healthy choice.*

STRAWBERRY BASIL QUENCHER

Calories: 30 kCal | Protein: 1 g | Carbohydrates: 8 g | Sugar: 5 g | Fat: 0,2 g | Fiber: 2 g | Cholesterol: 0 mg | Sodium: 15 mg | Phosphorus: 15 mg | Potassium: 110 mg.

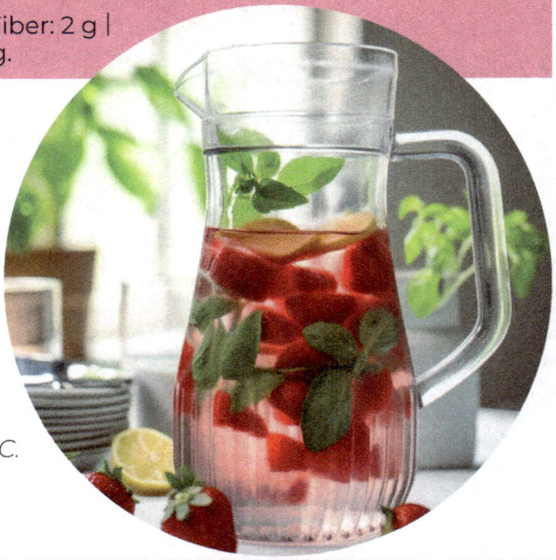

4 min | 10 min | 4

INGREDIENTS:

- 2 cups fresh strawberries, hulled and halved
- Ten fresh basil leaves
- 4 cups sparkling water
- One lemon, juiced

DIRECTIONS:

1. Basil and strawberries should be mixed in a pitcher's bottom.
2. Add lemon juice and sparkling water.
3. Stir gently, and serve over ice.

Heart-Healthy Benefits: *Strawberries offer antioxidants and vitamin C. Basil provides anti-inflammatory benefits. Lemon assists in digestion and detoxification.*

COOLING WATERMELON & LIME SLUSH

Calories: 50 kCal | Protein: 1 g | Carbohydrates: 12 g | Sugar: 9 g | Fat: 0,2 g | Fiber: 0,5 g | Cholesterol: 0 mg | Sodium: 3 mg | Phosphorus: 10 mg | Potassium: 170 mg.

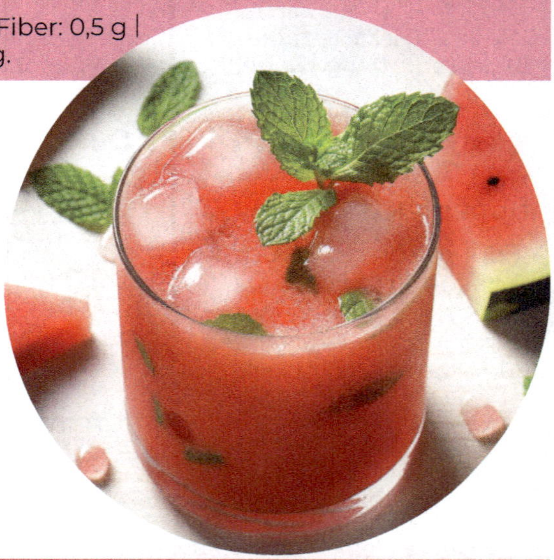

4 min | 10 min | 4

INGREDIENTS:

- 4 cups cubed watermelon, frozen
- Juice of 2 limes
- 1 tbsp agave nectar or honey
- 1/2 cup cold water

DIRECTIONS:

1. Combine frozen watermelon cubes, lime juice, agave nectar, and water in a blender.
2. Blend until smooth and slushy-like.
3. Serve immediately in chilled glasses.

Heart-Healthy Benefits: *Lycopene, associated with a lower risk of heart disease, is one of watermelon's many vitamins, minerals, and antioxidants.*

CREAMY AVOCADO & SPINACH SMOOTHIE

Calories: 190 kCal | Protein: 5 g | Carbohydrates: 12 g | Sugar: 4 g | Fat: 14 g | Fiber: 8 g | Cholesterol: 0 mg | Sodium: 80 mg | Phosphorus: 60 mg | Potassium: 450 mg.

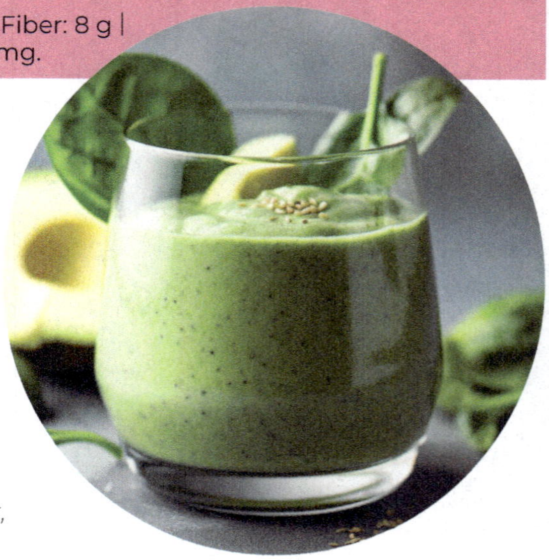

7 min | 0 min | 2

INGREDIENTS:

- One ripe avocado, peeled and pitted
- 1 cup fresh spinach leaves
- 2 cups almond milk (unsweetened)
- 1 tbsp chia seeds
- 1 tsp honey or agave nectar (optional)

DIRECTIONS:

1. Combine avocado, spinach, almond milk, chia seeds, and honey (if using) in a blender.
2. Blend until smooth and creamy.
3. Pour into glasses and serve immediately.

Heart-Healthy Benefits: *Monounsaturated fats, suitable for the heart, are abundant in avocados. At the same time, spinach offers many vitamins and minerals.*

POMEGRANATE GREEN TEA FUSION

Calories: 30 kCal | Protein: 0 g | Carbohydrates: 7 g | Sugar: 6 g | Fat: 0 g | Fiber: 0,5 g | Cholesterol: 0 mg | Sodium: 5 mg | Phosphorus: 10 mg | Potassium: 75 mg.

5 min | 3 min | 2

INGREDIENTS:

- Two green tea bags
- 2 cups boiling water
- 1/2 cup pomegranate juice, no added sugar
- Fresh pomegranate seeds for garnish

DIRECTIONS:

1. Steep green tea bags in boiling water for 3 minutes.
2. Remove tea bags and mix in pomegranate juice.
3. Garnish with fresh pomegranate seeds.
4. Serve warm or chilled.

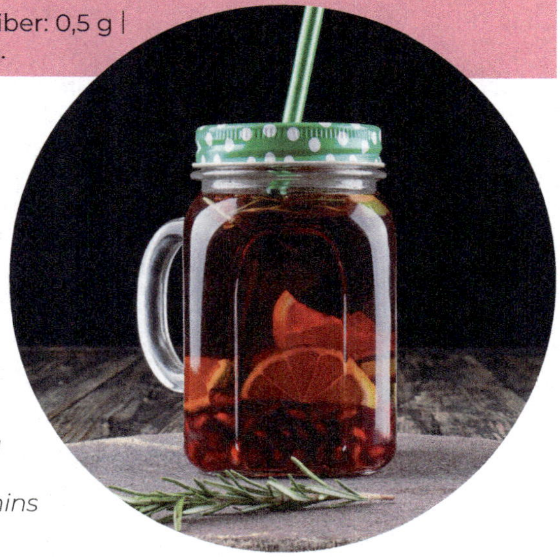

Heart-Healthy Benefits: *The potent antioxidant content of green tea is well known for its ability to decrease inflammation. Pomegranates contain powerful antioxidants known as punicalagin and anthocyanins that support heart health.*

MANGO & CHIA SEED REFRESHMENT

Calories: 70 kCal | Protein: 2 g | Carbohydrates: 15 g | Sugar: 13 g | Fat: 1 g | Fiber: 3 g | Cholesterol: 0 mg | Sodium: 5 mg | Phosphorus: 20 mg | Potassium: 210 mg.

15 min | 0 min | 4
(requires a few hours of chilling)

INGREDIENTS:

- Two ripe mangoes peeled and pitted
- 4 cups cold water
- 2 tbsp chia seeds
- 1 tbsp honey (optional)

DIRECTIONS:

1. In a blender, puree the mangoes with water until smooth.
2. Pour the mixture into a pitcher and stir in chia seeds.
3. Let the refreshment chill in the refrigerator for at least 2 hours to allow the chia seeds to expand.
4. Stir again before serving. Sweeten with honey if desired.

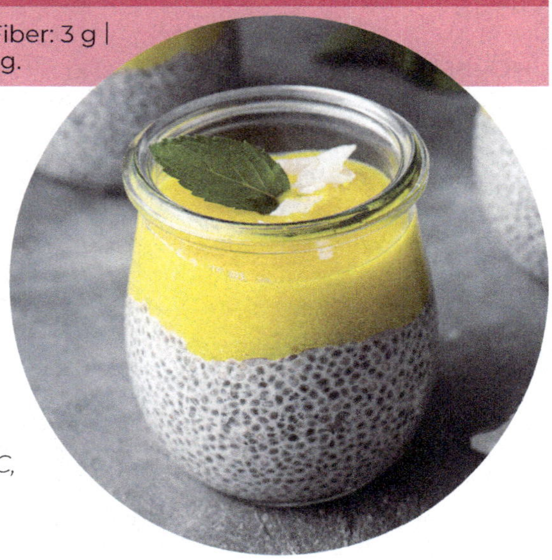

Heart-Healthy Benefits: *Mangoes provide dietary fiber and vitamin C, supporting heart health.*

NOTES

HEART-HEALTHY COCOA WITH A HINT OF CINNAMON

Calories: 60 kCal | Protein: 2 g | Carbohydrates: 10 g | Sugar: 6 g | Fat: 2,5 g | Fiber: 3 g | Cholesterol: 0 mg | Sodium: 180 mg | Phosphorus: 55 mg | Potassium: 240 mg.

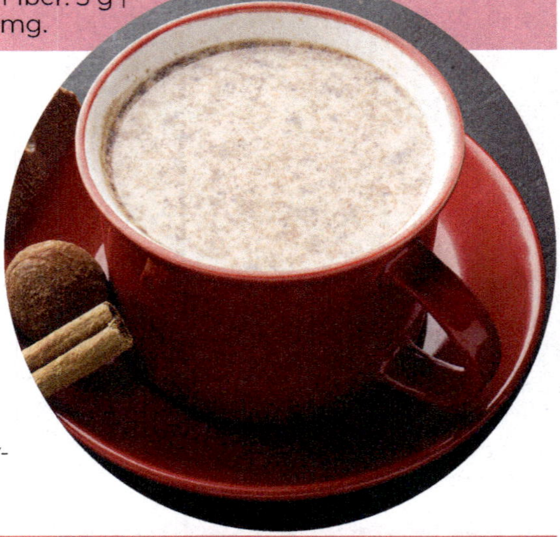

5 min | 10 min | 4

INGREDIENTS:

- 4 cups unsweetened almond milk
- 3 tbsp unsweetened cocoa powder
- 2 tbsp honey (or to taste)
- ½ tsp ground cinnamon

DIRECTIONS:

1. In a saucepan, heat the almond milk over medium heat.
2. Whisk in the cocoa powder until well combined.
3. Stir in honey and cinnamon.
4. Heat until warm but not boiling.
5. Serve in mugs.

Heart-Healthy Benefits: *Cocoa contains flavonoids, which are known to have heart-protective effects. Almond milk is a low-calorie and low-sodium alternative to dairy, making it a heart-friendly option.*

SOOTHING FENNEL & APPLE DRINK

Calories: 40 kCal | Protein: 0 g | Carbohydrates: 11 g | Sugar: 8 g | Fat: 0 g | Fiber: 2 g | Cholesterol: 0 mg | Sodium: 5 mg | Phosphorus: 10 mg | Potassium: 115 mg.

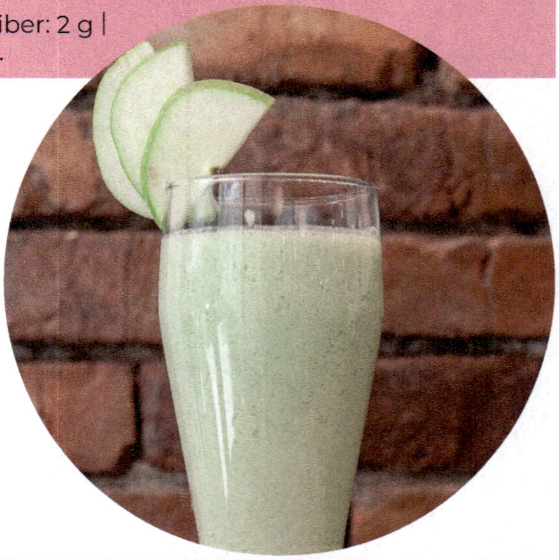

10 min | 5 min | 4

INGREDIENTS:

- Two green apples, sliced
- 1 tbsp fennel seeds
- 4 cups cold water

DIRECTIONS:

1. In a pitcher, combine apple slices and fennel seeds.
2. Fill with cold water and stir.
3. Refrigerate for at least 2 hours to infuse flavors.
4. Serve chilled.

Heart-Healthy Benefits: *Apples are a fantastic source of heart-healthy polyphenol antioxidants and dietary fiber. Fennel seeds may have properties that reduce blood pressure.*

CELERY & APPLE CLEANSE JUICE

Calories: 45 kCal | Protein: 1 g | Carbohydrates: 11 g | Sugar: 9 g | Fat: 0 g | Fiber: 2 g | Cholesterol: 0 mg | Sodium: 65 mg | Phosphorus: 20 mg | Potassium: 140 mg.

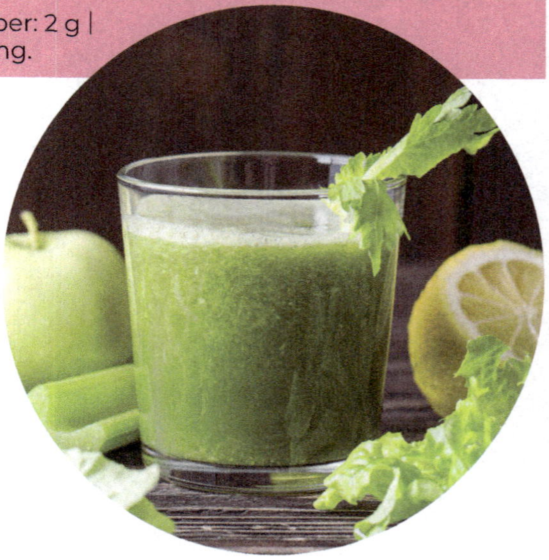

15 min | 0 min | 2

INGREDIENTS:

- Three celery stalks
- Two green apples, cored
- One lemon, juiced
- 1-inch piece of fresh ginger

DIRECTIONS:

5. Wash and chop the celery and apples.
6. Use a juicer to extract the juice from the celery, apples, and ginger.
7. Stir in the lemon juice.
8. Serve immediately over ice.

Heart-Healthy Benefits: *Celery contains phthalides, which may help lower high blood pressure. Apples are a great source of dietary fiber and heart-healthy antioxidants.*

BANANA & WALNUT MUFFINS

Calories: 185 kCal | Protein: 4 g | Carbohydrates: 38 g | Sugar: 17 g | Fat: 3,5 g | Fiber: 4 g | Cholesterol: 0 mg | Sodium: 105 mg | Phosphorus: 60 mg | Potassium: 250 mg.

15 min | 20 min | 6

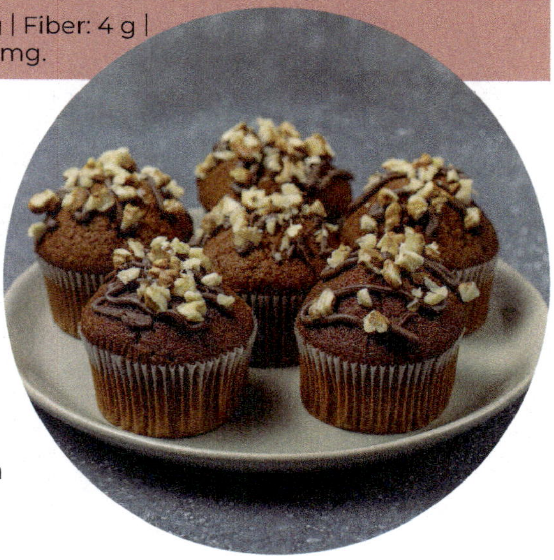

Ingredients:

- Two ripe bananas, mashed
- 1/4 cup almond milk
- 1/4 cup maple syrup
- 1 cup whole wheat flour
- 1/2 tsp baking soda
- 1/4 cup chopped walnuts
- Pinch of salt

Directions:

1. Preheat the oven to 375°F (190°C).
2. Combine mashed bananas, almond milk, and maple syrup in a mixing bowl.
3. Whisk together whole wheat flour, baking soda, and salt in another bowl.
4. Fold the dry ingredients into the wet mixture until just combined.
5. Stir in the chopped walnuts.
6. Divide the batter among six muffin tins.
7. Bake for 20 minutes or until a toothpick inserted comes out clean.
8. Allow the muffins to cool on a wire rack.

Heart-Healthy Benefits: *Whole wheat flour offers more nutrients and fiber than refined flour. Walnuts provide omega-3 fatty acids, which are known for their cardiovascular benefits. Bananas add natural sweetness and potassium, which is beneficial for heart health.*

OATMEAL & RAISIN COOKIES

Calories: 150 kCal | Protein: 3 g | Carbohydrates: 25 g | Sugar: 11 g | Fat: 5 g | Fiber: 3 g | Cholesterol: 0 mg | Sodium: 50 mg | Phosphorus: 30 mg | Potassium: 180 mg.

15 min | 15 min | 6

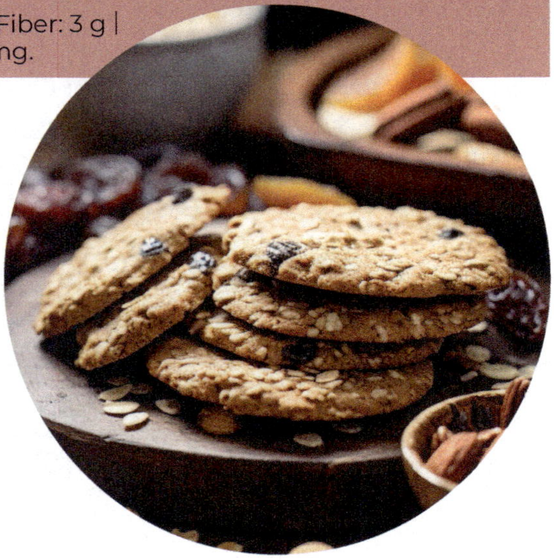

Ingredients:

- 1 cup rolled oats
- 1/2 cup raisins
- 1/4 cup almond butter
- 2 tbsp maple syrup
- 1 tsp vanilla extract
- 1/2 tsp baking soda
- 1/4 tsp cinnamon
- Pinch of salt

Directions:

1. Preheat the oven to 350°F (175°C) and line a baking tray with parchment paper.
2. Combine rolled oats, raisins, almond butter, maple syrup, and vanilla extract in a large bowl.
3. Add in baking soda, cinnamon, and salt. Mix until well combined.
4. Using your hands, shape the mixture into small cookie-sized balls and place them on the prepared tray.
5. Flatten each ball slightly with a fork.
6. Bake for 12-15 minutes or until golden brown.
7. Allow the cookies to cool on the tray before transferring them to a wire rack.

Heart-Healthy Benefits: *Oats are known to lower harmful cholesterol levels, thus benefiting heart health. Raisins offer antioxidants and fiber. Almond butter provides heart-healthy monounsaturated fats. This recipe avoids refined sugars by utilizing the natural sweetness of maple syrup.*

FLUFFY PUMPKIN PANCAKES

Calories: 210 kCal | Protein: 6 g | Carbohydrates: 46 g | Sugar: 8 g | Fat: 2 g | Fiber: 7 g | Cholesterol: 0 mg | Sodium: 150 mg | Phosphorus: 110 mg | Potassium: 245 mg.

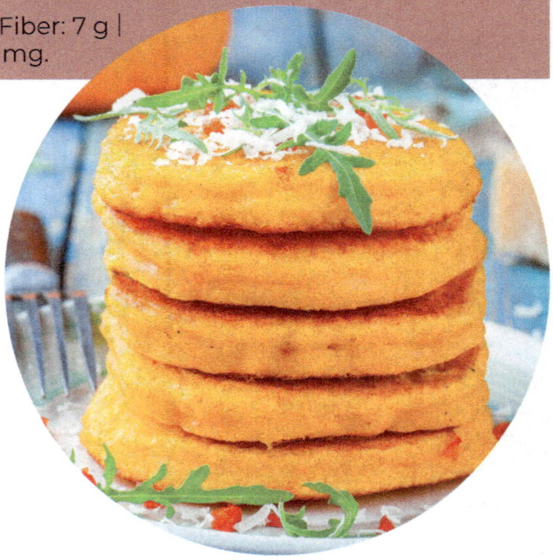

15 min | 20 min | 6

Ingredients:

- 1 cup pumpkin puree
- 1 1/2 cups almond milk
- 2 tsp vanilla extract
- 2 cups whole wheat flour
- 2 tsp baking powder
- 1/4 tsp ground cinnamon
- 1/4 tsp ground nutmeg
- Pinch of salt
- Maple syrup for serving

Directions:

1. Combine the pumpkin puree, almond milk, and vanilla extract in a mixing bowl.
2. Sift together the whole wheat flour, baking powder, cinnamon, nutmeg, and salt in another bowl.
3. Gradually add the dry mixture to the wet ingredients, stirring until combined.
4. Heat a non-stick skillet over medium heat.
5. Pour 1/4 cup batter for each pancake and cook until bubbles form on the surface. Flip and cook until the other side is golden brown.
6. Serve with a drizzle of maple syrup.

Heart-Healthy Benefits: *Antioxidants, vitamins, and minerals found in pumpkins are suitable for the heart. Whole wheat flour has a lot of dietary fiber, reducing heart disease risk. Saturated fats and cholesterol are absent from almond milk.*

CRANBERRY ALMOND SCONES

Calories: 260 kCal | Protein: 7 g | Carbohydrates: 47 g | Sugar: 14 g | Fat: 7 g | Fiber: 6 g | Cholesterol: 0 mg | Sodium: 80 mg | Phosphorus: 135 mg | Potassium: 200 mg.

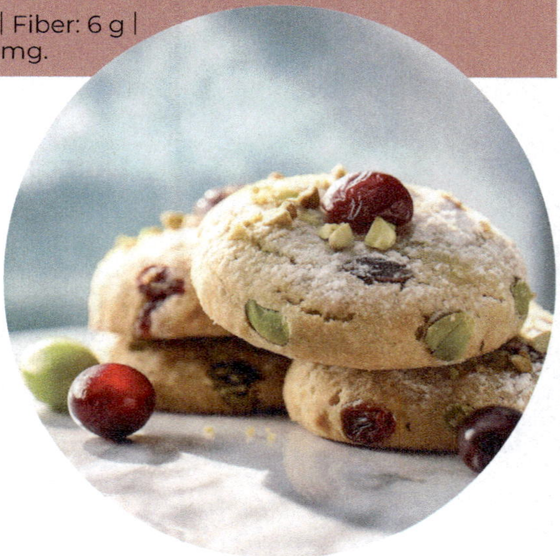

15 min | 20 min | 6

Ingredients:

- 2 cups whole wheat flour
- 1/4 cup maple syrup
- 1/2 cup almond milk
- 1/4 cup chopped almonds
- 1/2 cup dried cranberries
- 2 tsp baking powder
- 1/4 tsp salt
- 2 tbsp coconut oil, solid

Directions:

1. Preheat the oven to 400°F (200°C) and line a baking sheet with parchment paper.
2. Combine whole wheat flour, baking powder, and salt in a bowl.
3. Cut in the solid coconut oil until the mixture resembles coarse crumbs.
4. Add maple syrup, almond milk, chopped almonds, and dried cranberries. Mix until just combined.
5. Shape the dough into an 8-inch circle on a floured surface and cut into six wedges.
6. Place the wedges on the prepared baking sheet and bake for 18-20 minutes or until golden brown.

Heart-Healthy Benefits: *Cranberries are known for their antioxidants, which can decrease blood pressure and increase good cholesterol. Almonds contain healthy fats and vitamin E, which help maintain a healthy heart. Although it has saturated fats, coconut oil contains a type that's considered more beneficial and can have a neutral impact on cholesterol.*

LEMON POPPY SEED CAKE

Calories: 265 kCal | Protein: 8 g | Carbohydrates: 30 g | Sugar: 15 g | Fat: 15 g | Fiber: 4 g | Cholesterol: 0 mg | Sodium: 70 mg | Phosphorus: 120 mg | Potassium: 250 mg.

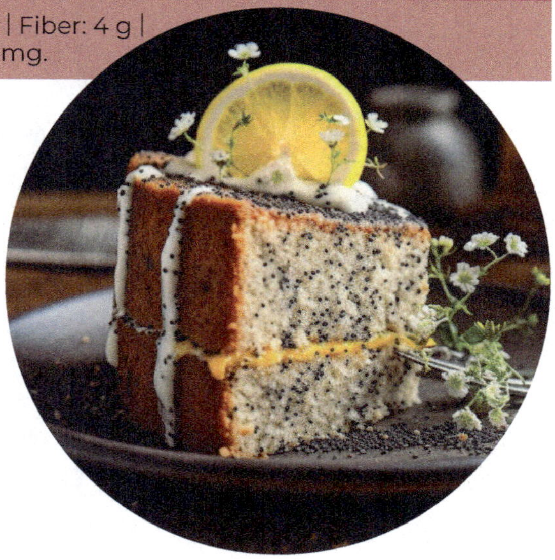

15 min | 30 min | 4

INGREDIENTS:

- 1 1/2 cups almond flour
- 1/2 cup maple syrup
- 2 tsp lemon zest
- 3 tbsp lemon juice
- 2 tbsp poppy seeds
- 2 tsp baking powder
- 1/4 tsp salt
- 1/4 cup almond milk

DIRECTIONS:

1. Preheat the oven to 350°F (175°C) and line a loaf pan with parchment paper.
2. Combine almond flour, maple syrup, lemon zest, lemon juice, poppy seeds, baking powder, and salt in a large mixing bowl.
3. Gradually add almond milk, mixing until the batter is smooth.
4. Pour the batter into the prepared pan and spread evenly.
5. Bake for 25-30 minutes or until a toothpick inserted in the center comes clean.
6. Allow to cool before removing from the pan and slicing.

Heart-Healthy Benefits: *Almonds are packed with monounsaturated fats, which can help reduce heart disease risks. Lemons are rich in vitamin C, known for its heart-protecting effects. Poppy seeds provide dietary fiber and essential nutrients beneficial for heart health.*

APPLE SPICE BUNDT CAKE

Calories: 275 kCal | Protein: 6 g | Carbohydrates: 48 g | Sugar: 18 g | Fat: 8 g | Fiber: 5 g | Cholesterol: 0 mg | Sodium: 90 mg | Phosphorus: 180 mg | Potassium: 280 mg.

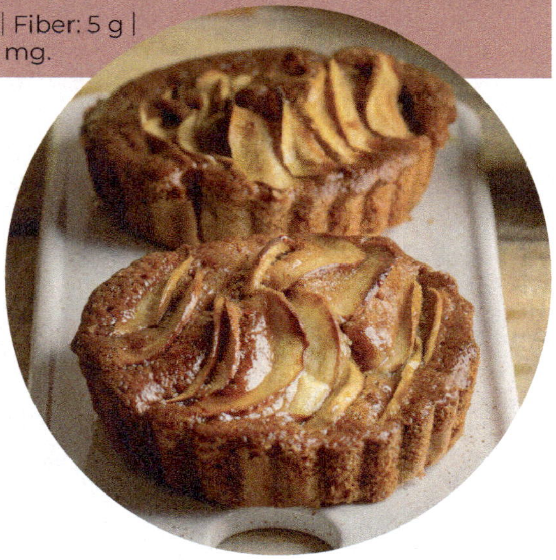

20 min | 35 min | 6

INGREDIENTS:

- 2 cups whole wheat flour
- 2 tsp baking powder
- 1 tsp ground cinnamon
- 1/2 tsp ground nutmeg
- 1/4 tsp ground cloves
- 1/4 tsp salt
- Two large apples, peeled, cored, and grated
- 1/2 cup maple syrup
- 1/3 cup almond milk
- 1/4 cup coconut oil, melted
- 2 tsp vanilla extract

DIRECTIONS:

1. Preheat the oven to 350°F (175°C) and grease a Bundt pan.
2. Whisk together whole wheat flour, baking powder, cinnamon, nutmeg, cloves, and salt in a large bowl.
3. Combine grated apples, maple syrup, almond milk, melted coconut oil, and vanilla extract in another bowl.
4. Mix the wet ingredients into the dry ingredients until just combined.
5. Pour the batter into the prepared Bundt pan, smoothing out the top.
6. Bake for 30-35 minutes or until a skewer comes out clean when inserted.
7. Let it cool for about 10 minutes, then turn it onto a wire rack to cool completely.

Heart-Healthy Benefits: *Whole wheat flour provides dietary fiber that can help lower cholesterol. Apples are high in antioxidants, particularly quercetin, beneficial for heart health. Spices like cinnamon can positively affect heart health due to their anti-inflammatory properties.*

VANILLA BEAN PUDDING WITH FRESH BERRIES

Calories: 130 kCal | Protein: 2 g | Carbohydrates: 30 g | Sugar: 20 g | Fat: 1,5 g | Fiber: 2 g | Cholesterol: 0 mg | Sodium: 40 mg | Phosphorus: 50 mg | Potassium: 180 mg.

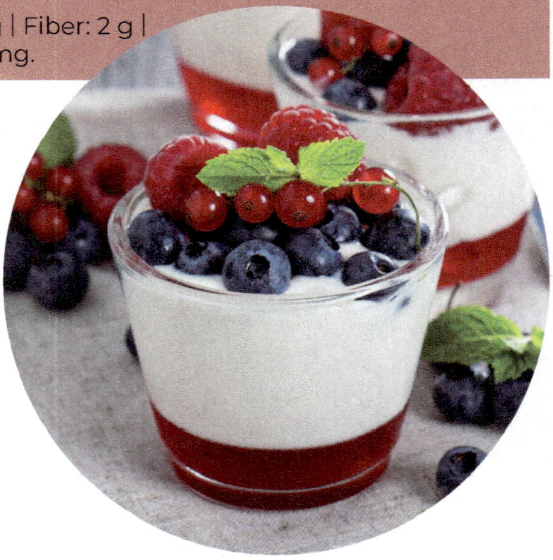

10 min | 10 min | 4
(plus chilling time)

INGREDIENTS:

- 2 cups unsweetened almond milk
- 1/4 cup cornstarch
- 1/3 cup maple syrup
- One vanilla bean, split, and seeds scraped
- 1 cup mixed fresh berries (blueberries, raspberries, strawberries)

DIRECTIONS:

1. In a saucepan, whisk together almond milk and cornstarch until smooth.
2. Add maple syrup and the seeds from the vanilla bean to the saucepan.
3. Cook over medium heat, stirring constantly until the mixture thickens to a pudding consistency.
4. Remove from heat and transfer the pudding to individual serving dishes.
5. Chill in the refrigerator for at least 2 hours.
6. Before serving, top each pudding with fresh berries.

Heart-Healthy Benefits: *Berries are packed with antioxidants and dietary fiber that can promote heart health. Magnesium and vitamin E, two nutrients that can strengthen arteries and lower the risk of heart disease, are abundant in almond milk.*

DARK CHOCOLATE & AVOCADO TRUFFLES

Calories: 220 kCal | Protein: 3 g | Carbohydrates: 18 g | Sugar: 8 g | Fat: 15 g | Fiber: 7 g | Cholesterol: 0 mg | Sodium: 60 mg | Phosphorus: 90 mg | Potassium: 320 mg.

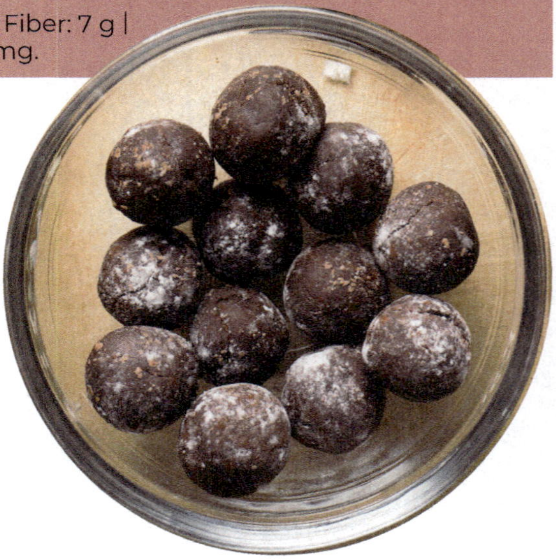

20 min | 0 min | 6
(chill time: 2 hours)

INGREDIENTS:

- One ripe avocado, pitted and mashed
- 3.5 oz dark chocolate (at least 70% cacao), melted
- 1 tsp vanilla extract
- A pinch of sea salt
- Unsweetened cocoa powder for dusting

DIRECTIONS:

1. In a mixing bowl, combine mashed avocado and melted dark chocolate. Mix until smooth.
2. Stir in vanilla extract and sea salt.
3. Chill the mixture in the refrigerator for about 30 minutes.
4. Once chilled, shape the mixture into small balls.
5. Roll each ball in cocoa powder to coat.
6. Place the truffles back in the refrigerator for another 30 minutes to set.
7. Serve chilled.

Heart-Healthy Benefits: *Dark chocolate includes flavonoids that may increase blood flow and lower blood pressure, particularly those with a more fantastic cacao content. Avocados provide healthy monounsaturated fats, which can benefit heart health.*

NOTES

CHERRY & OAT CRUMBLE BARS

Calories: 210 kCal | Protein: 5 g | Carbohydrates: 40 g | Sugar: 12 g | Fat: 6 g | Fiber: 5 g | Cholesterol: 0 mg | Sodium: 30 mg | Phosphorus: 70 mg | Potassium: 210 mg.

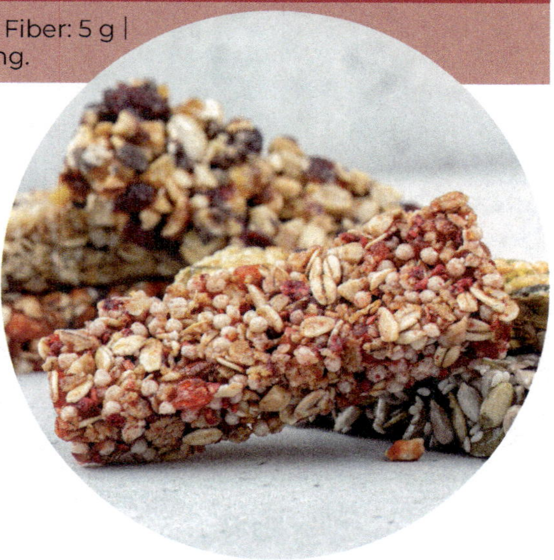

20 min | 35 min | 4

Ingredients:

- 2 cups fresh cherries, pitted and chopped
- 1 cup rolled oats
- 1/2 cup whole wheat flour
- 1/3 cup pure maple syrup
- 1/4 cup almond butter
- 1 tsp vanilla extract
- 1/4 tsp almond extract
- A pinch of sea salt

Directions:

1. Preheat the oven to 350°F (175°C) and line an 8x8-inch baking dish with parchment paper.
2. Combine oats, whole wheat flour, maple syrup, almond butter, vanilla extract, almond extract, and sea salt in a mixing bowl.
3. Press half of the mixture firmly into the bottom of the prepared baking dish.
4. Layer with chopped cherries.
5. Sprinkle the remaining oat mixture over the cherries and press gently.
6. Bake for 30-35 minutes or until golden brown. Allow to cool before cutting into bars.

Heart-Healthy Benefits: *Anthocyanins, which are abundant in cherries and have antioxidant characteristics, may help lessen inflammation. Oats contain beta-glucans, a soluble fiber that can help lower cholesterol levels.*

WHOLE WHEAT CHOCOLATE CHIP COOKIES

Calories: 180 kCal | Protein: 4 g | Carbohydrates: 24 g | Sugar: 12 g | Fat: 8 g | Fiber: 3 g | Cholesterol: 30 mg | Sodium: 50 mg | Phosphorus: 60 mg | Potassium: 80 mg.

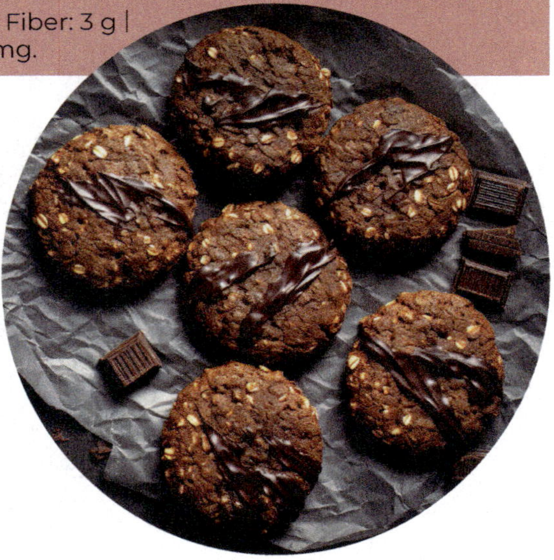

20 min | 12 min | 6

Ingredients:

- 1 cup whole wheat flour
- 1/2 tsp baking soda
- 1/4 cup coconut oil, melted
- 1/4 cup maple syrup
- One egg
- 1 tsp vanilla extract
- 1/3 cup dark chocolate chips (at least 70% cocoa)

Directions:

1. Preheat the oven to 350°F (175°C) and line a baking sheet with parchment paper.
2. In a bowl, combine whole wheat flour and baking soda.
3. Whisk together coconut oil, maple syrup, egg, and vanilla extract in another bowl.
4. Gradually mix the wet ingredients into the dry, then fold the chocolate chips.
5. Spoonfuls of dough should be dropped and slightly flattened on the baking sheet.
6. Bake for 10-12 minutes or until golden. Allow to cool on the baking sheet.

Heart-Healthy Benefits: *Dark chocolate (especially 70% cocoa or higher) contains flavonoids, which have been shown to have heart-protective qualities. Whole wheat flour adds dietary fiber, which can help lower cholesterol and improve heart health.*

APPLE & GINGERBREAD UPSIDE-DOWN CAKE

Calories: 250 kCal | Protein: 5 g | Carbohydrates: 38 g | Sugar: 19 g | Fat: 9 g | Fiber: 4 g | Cholesterol: 60 mg | Sodium: 150 mg | Phosphorus: 90 mg | Potassium: 180 mg.

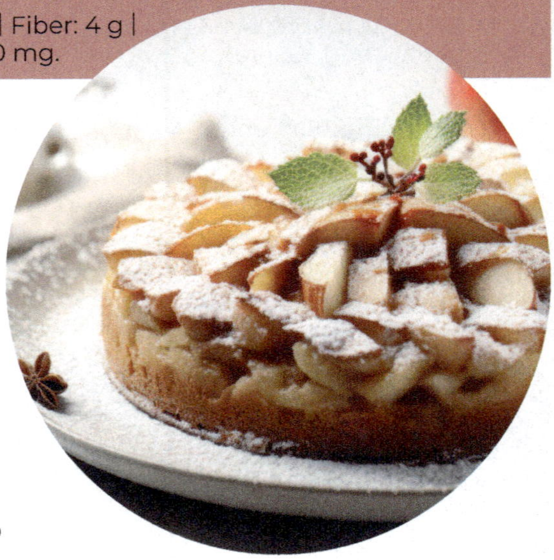

25 min | 35 min | 6

INGREDIENTS:

- Two ripe apples, thinly sliced
- 1/4 cup honey or maple syrup divided
- 1 1/2 cups whole wheat flour
- 1 tsp baking soda
- 2 tsp ground ginger
- 1 tsp ground cinnamon
- 1/4 tsp ground cloves
- 1/4 cup molasses
- 1/4 cup apple sauce
- 1/4 cup olive oil or coconut oil
- Two eggs
- 1 tsp vanilla extract

DIRECTIONS:

1. Preheat the oven to 350°F (175°C). Grease a round cake pan and arrange the apple slices at the bottom. Drizzle with half of the honey or maple syrup.
2. Whisk together flour, baking soda, ginger, cinnamon, and cloves in a bowl.
3. Combine molasses, remaining honey or maple syrup, apple sauce, oil, eggs, and vanilla in another bowl.
4. Gradually fold the wet mixture into the dry mix until well combined.
5. Pour the batter over the apples, spreading it evenly.
6. Bake for 30-35 minutes or until a toothpick comes out clean. Allow to cool before inverting onto a plate.

Heart-Healthy Benefits: *Dietary fiber, abundant in pears, may help lower cholesterol levels. Ginger has anti-inflammatory properties, which can be beneficial for heart health. Whole wheat flour provides essential nutrients and fiber beneficial for cardiovascular health.*

SATISFYING YOUR SWEET TOOTH THE HEART-HEALTHY WAY

DARK CHOCOLATE-DIPPED STRAWBERRIES

Calories: 150 kCal | Protein: 3 g | Carbohydrates: 20 g | Sugar: 14 g | Fat: 7 g | Fiber: 3 g | Cholesterol: 0 mg | Sodium: 5 mg | Phosphorus: 40 mg | Potassium: 180 mg.

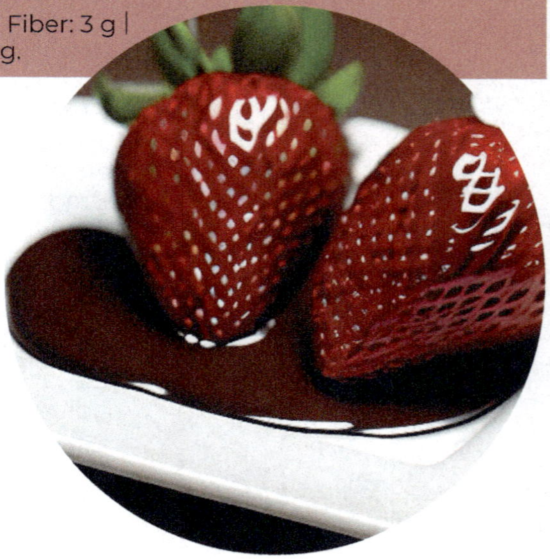

15 min | 5 min | 4

INGREDIENTS:

- 1 pint fresh strawberries, washed and dried
- 3/4 cup dark chocolate (70% cocoa or higher), roughly chopped

DIRECTIONS:

1. Line a baking sheet with parchment paper.
2. Melt dark chocolate in a heatproof bowl set over a pan of simmering water, stirring occasionally.
3. Once melted, dip each strawberry into the chocolate, covering about half to three-quarters of the strawberry.
4. Place each dipped strawberry on the parchment paper.
5. Chill in the refrigerator for at least 1 hour or until the chocolate is set.

Heart-Healthy Benefits: *Dark chocolate is loaded with flavonoids, which are beneficial for heart health. Strawberries provide essential vitamins, fiber, and antioxidants beneficial for cardiovascular health.*

CREAMY AVOCADO & CHOCOLATE MOUSSE

Calories: 220 kCal | Protein: 4 g | Carbohydrates: 30 g | Sugar: 18 g | Fat: 12 g | Fiber: 8 g | Cholesterol: 0 mg | Sodium: 10 mg | Phosphorus: 60 mg | Potassium: 500 mg.

20 min | 35 min | 4

INGREDIENTS:

- Two ripe avocados, pitted and scooped
- 1/2 cup unsweetened cocoa powder
- 1/4 cup honey or maple syrup
- 1 tsp vanilla extract
- A pinch of sea salt
- Fresh berries for garnish

DIRECTIONS:

1. Combine avocados, cocoa powder, honey or maple syrup, vanilla extract, and sea salt in a blender or food processor. Blend until smooth and creamy.
2. Transfer the mousse to individual serving dishes.
3. Chill in the refrigerator for at least 2 hours before serving.
4. Garnish with fresh berries before serving.

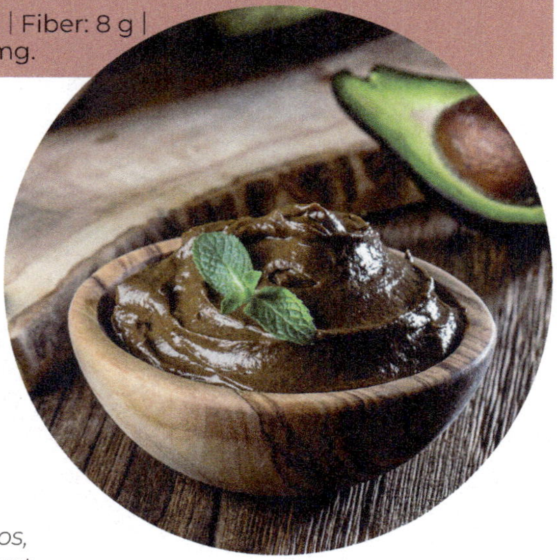

Heart-Healthy Benefits: *Monounsaturated fats, abundant in avocados, may help lower dangerous cholesterol levels and lessen the risk of heart disease. The unsweetened cocoa powder provides flavonoids beneficial for heart health.*

COCONUT & MATCHA ENERGY BALLS

Calories: 190 kCal | Protein: 3 g | Carbohydrates: 23 g | Sugar: 18 g | Fat: 11 g | Fiber: 6 g | Cholesterol: 0 mg | Sodium: 10 mg | Phosphorus: 50 mg | Potassium: 80 mg.

20 min | 0 min | 4

INGREDIENTS:

- 1 cup unsweetened shredded coconut, plus extra for rolling
- 1/4 cup chia seeds
- 1 tbsp matcha green tea powder
- 1/4 cup honey or maple syrup
- 1 tsp vanilla extract

DIRECTIONS:

1. Combine shredded coconut, chia seeds, and matcha powder in a mixing bowl.
2. Add honey and vanilla extract, mixing until a sticky mixture forms.
3. Roll the mixture into small balls, using about a tablespoon for each.
4. Roll the balls in extra shredded coconut to coat.
5. Place on a parchment-lined tray and chill in the refrigerator for at least 1 hour before serving.

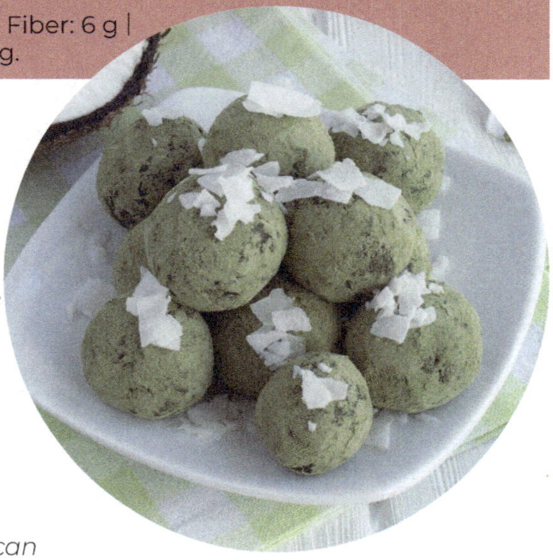

Heart-Healthy Benefits: *Antioxidants included in matcha green tea can help stop cell damage and lessen inflammation. Omega-3 fatty acids, thought to lower the risk of heart disease, are abundant in chia seeds.*

NOTES

BONUS: AIR FRYER RECIPES

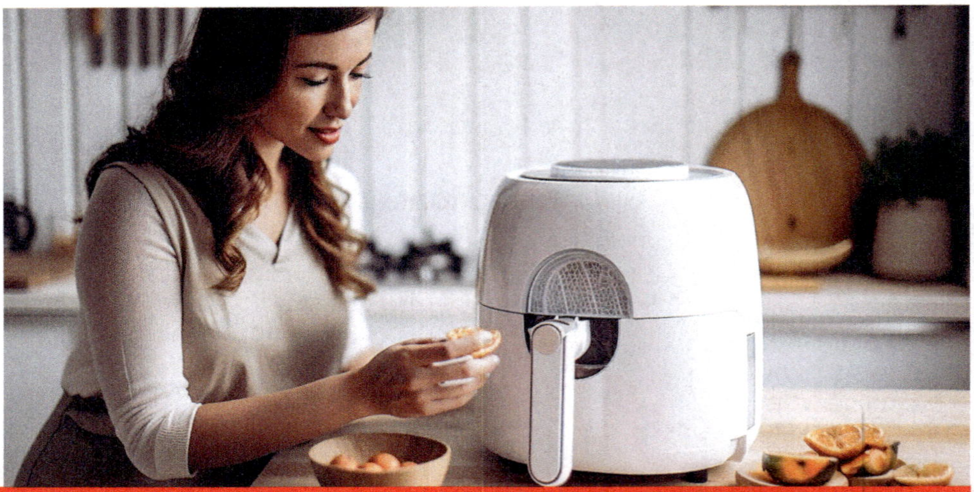

TERIYAKI GLAZED SALMON FILETS

Calories: 265 kCal | Protein: 28 g | Carbohydrates: 10 g | Sugar: 9 g | Fat: 11 g | Fiber: 0 g | Cholesterol: 60 mg | Sodium: 400 mg | Phosphorus: 310 mg | Potassium: 530 mg.

15 min | 12 min | 6 (plus marinating time)

INGREDIENTS:

- Four salmon filets (about four oz. each)
- 1/4 cup low-sodium soy sauce
- 2 tbsp honey
- 1 tbsp fresh ginger, grated
- Two cloves garlic, minced
- 1 tsp sesame oil
- Two green onions, sliced for garnish
- 1 tbsp sesame seeds for garnish

DIRECTIONS:

1. Mix the soy sauce, honey, ginger, garlic, and sesame oil in a mixing bowl to create the teriyaki marinade.
2. Place salmon filets in a shallow dish and pour marinade over them. Let marinate for at least 30 minutes in the refrigerator.
3. Preheat the air fryer to 400°F (205°C).
4. Place the marinated salmon filets in the air fryer and cook for 10-12 minutes or until the salmon flakes easily with a fork.
5. Serve hot, garnished with sliced green onions and a sprinkle of sesame seeds.

Heart-Healthy Benefits: *Omega-3 fatty acids, abundant in salmon, can reduce inflammation, blood pressure, and disease risk factors. Soy sauce and sesame provide beneficial compounds that can improve heart health, but use them in moderation due to their sodium content.*

HERBED CORN ON THE COB

Calories: 280 kCal | Protein: 12 g | Carbohydrates: 36 g | Sugar: 4 g | Fat: 10 g | Fiber: 4 g | Cholesterol: 25 mg | Sodium: 300 mg | Phosphorus: 140 mg | Potassium: 380 mg.

10 min | 10 min | 4

INGREDIENTS:

- Four years of corn-husked
- 2 tbsp olive oil
- 1 tsp dried rosemary
- 1 tsp dried thyme
- Salt to taste (keep sodium below 20% of daily intake)
- Freshly ground black pepper

DIRECTIONS:

1. Preheat the air fryer to 400°F (205°C).
2. Mix olive oil, rosemary, thyme, salt, and black pepper in a small bowl.
3. Brush the corn ears with the herb and oil mixture.
4. Place the corn in the air fryer and cook for about 12 minutes, turning halfway through or until the kernels are tender.
5. Serve hot.

Heart-Healthy Benefits: *Corn provides beneficial fiber, which can help lower cholesterol levels in the blood. Monounsaturated fats and antioxidants found in olive oil help reduce the risk of cardiovascular disease.*

SPINACH AND FETA STUFFED CHICKEN BREAST

Calories: 230 kCal | Protein: 30 g | Carbohydrates: 3 g | Sugar: 1 g | Fat: 11 g | Fiber: 1 g | Cholesterol: 85 mg | Sodium: 250 mg | Phosphorus: 220 mg | Potassium: 380 mg.

10 min | 20 min | 4

Ingredients:

- Four boneless, skinless chicken breasts
- 1 cup fresh spinach, chopped
- 1/2 cup feta cheese, crumbled (use low-fat version if available)
- 1 tbsp olive oil
- Two cloves garlic, minced
- Salt to taste (keep sodium below 20% of daily intake)
- Freshly ground black pepper
- 1 tsp dried oregano

Directions:

1. Preheat the air fryer to 380°F (193°C).
2. In a small pan, heat olive oil and sauté garlic until fragrant. Add spinach and cook until wilted. Remove from heat and mix in feta cheese.
3. Create a pocket in each chicken breast by slicing it into the thickest part without cutting it through. Stuff each bag with the spinach and feta mixture.
4. Season the outside of the chicken breasts with a pinch of salt, pepper, and oregano.
5. Place the chicken breasts in the air fryer and cook for about 20 minutes or until the chicken is fully cooked.
6. Serve hot.

Heart-Healthy Benefits: *Chicken provides lean protein essential for muscle health. Spinach is a good source of dietary nitrates, which can help decrease blood pressure and improve heart health. Feta, while flavorful, is used in moderation to control sodium and fat intake.*

PARMESAN & HERB ZUCCHINI STICKS

Calories: 280 kCal | Protein: 12 g | Carbohydrates: 36 g | Sugar: 4 g | Fat: 10 g | Fiber: 4 g | Cholesterol: 25 mg | Sodium: 300 mg | Phosphorus: 140 mg | Potassium: 380 mg.

10 min | 10 min | 4

Ingredients:

- Four whole-grain mini pizza crusts
- 1 cup low-sodium tomato sauce
- 1 cup shredded mozzarella cheese (opt for low-fat)
- 1 cup cherry tomatoes, halved
- Fresh basil leaves
- Olive oil for drizzling
- Salt to taste (keep sodium below 20% of daily intake)

Directions:

1. Preheat the air fryer to 375°F (190°C).
2. Spread a layer of tomato sauce over each mini pizza crust.
3. Sprinkle mozzarella cheese evenly over the sauce.
4. Top with cherry tomato halves.
5. Place the mini pizzas in the air fryer, in batches if necessary, and cook for about 10 minutes or until the cheese is melted and bubbly.
6. Remove from the air fryer, drizzle with olive oil, sprinkle a pinch of salt, and top with fresh basil leaves.
7. Serve immediately.

Heart-Healthy Benefits: *Whole grains promote heart health by lowering the risk of heart disease and raising blood cholesterol levels. Lycopene, a powerful antioxidant linked to a lower risk of heart disease, is abundant in tomatoes. The use of low-sodium ingredients ensures that sodium intake remains controlled.*

NOTES

GOLDEN AIR-FRIED POTATOES WITH ROSEMARY

Calories: 220 kCal | Protein: 4 g | Carbohydrates: 40 g | Sugar: 3 g | Fat: 5 g | Fiber: 3 g | Cholesterol: 0 mg | Sodium: 80 mg | Phosphorus: 75 mg | Potassium: 900 mg.

10 min | 20 min | 4

INGREDIENTS:

- Four medium russet potatoes sliced into wedges
- 2 tbsp olive oil
- 2 tsp fresh rosemary, chopped
- Salt to taste (keep sodium below 20% of daily intake)

DIRECTIONS:

1. Preheat the air fryer to 380°F (190°C).
2. Toss the potato wedges with olive oil, rosemary, and a pinch of salt in a large mixing bowl.
3. Place potato wedges in the air fryer in a single layer.
4. Cook for 20 minutes, shaking halfway through until the potatoes are golden brown and crisp.
5. Serve immediately.

Heart-Healthy Benefits: *Potatoes provide vitamin C, potassium, and fiber, especially if you eat the skin. Rosemary provides antioxidants.*

PARMESAN & HERB ZUCCHINI STICKS

Calories: 100 kCal | Protein: 4 g | Carbohydrates: 4 g | Sugar: 2 g | Fat: 8 g | Fiber: 1 g | Cholesterol: 5 mg | Sodium: 150 mg | Phosphorus: 40 mg | Potassium: 250 mg.

10 min | 12 min | 4

INGREDIENTS:

- Two medium zucchinis, cut into sticks
- 2 tbsp olive oil
- 1/4 cup grated parmesan cheese
- 2 tsp mixed dried herbs (like basil, oregano, and thyme)
- Salt to taste (keep sodium below 20% of daily intake)

DIRECTIONS:

1. Preheat the air fryer to 380°F (190°C).
2. Toss zucchini sticks with olive oil in a bowl.
3. Mix parmesan cheese, herbs, and a pinch of salt in another bowl.
4. Roll zucchini sticks in the cheese mixture until well coated.
5. Place in the air fryer in a single layer and cook for 12 minutes or until golden.
6. Serve with a dipping sauce of choice.

Heart-Healthy Benefits: *Zucchinis are a fantastic fiber and vitamin C source, which can lower cholesterol. Olive oil and parmesan provide healthy fats that can aid heart health. Herbs not only elevate the flavor but also have anti-inflammatory properties.*

SPICED CARROT FRIES

Calories: 90 kCal | Protein: 1 g | Carbohydrates: 10 g | Sugar: 5 g | Fat: 5 g | Fiber: 3 g | Cholesterol: 0 mg | Sodium: 70 mg | Phosphorus: 40 mg | Potassium: 370 mg.

10 min | 20 min | 4

INGREDIENTS:

- Four large carrots peeled and cut into fries-like shape
- 2 tbsp olive oil
- 1 tsp ground cumin
- 1/2 tsp smoked paprika
- Salt to taste (keep sodium below 20% of daily intake)

DIRECTIONS:

1. Preheat the air fryer to 375°F (190°C).
2. In a mixing bowl, toss the carrot fries with olive oil, cumin, paprika, and a pinch of salt.
3. Place carrot fries in the air fryer, ensuring they are spaced out and not overlapping.
4. Cook for 20 minutes, turning halfway through, until the carrots are crisp on the outside and tender inside.
5. Serve with a side of hummus or any low-sodium dip.

Heart-Healthy Benefits: *Because they are high in fiber, carrots can help decrease cholesterol levels. They also provide vitamin A and beta-carotene, which have heart-protective properties. Cumin and paprika are antioxidants, while olive oil is a source of beneficial monounsaturated fats.*

GARLIC PARMESAN GREEN BEANS

Calories: 110 kCal | Protein: 5 g | Carbohydrates: 11 g | Sugar: 3 g | Fat: 6 g | Fiber: 4 g | Cholesterol: 5 mg | Sodium: 180 mg | Phosphorus: 50 mg | Potassium: 239 mg.

10 min | 10 min | 4

INGREDIENTS:

- 1 lb fresh green beans, trimmed
- 2 tbsp olive oil
- Three cloves garlic, minced
- 1/4 cup grated Parmesan cheese (ensure plant-based or skip for vegan option)
- Salt to taste (keeping sodium below 20% of daily intake)
- Freshly ground black pepper
- Zest of 1 lemon

DIRECTIONS:

1. Toss the green beans with olive oil, minced garlic, salt, and black pepper in a large bowl.
2. Preheat the air fryer to 375°F (190°C).
3. Place the green beans in the air fryer basket and cook for about 10 minutes, shaking halfway through, until tender and slightly crispy.
4. Once done, place in a serving bowl and toss with lemon zest and Parmesan cheese.
5. Serve immediately.

Heart-Healthy Benefits: *Green beans are a low-calorie food that contains vitamins, minerals, and fiber. Olive oil provides heart-healthy fats, while garlic offers antioxidant properties beneficial for heart health.*

CINNAMON SUGAR BUTTERNUT SQUASH

Calories: 115 kCal | Protein: 1 g | Carbohydrates: 30 g | Sugar: 7 g | Fat: 4 g | Fiber: 5 g | Cholesterol: 0 mg | Sodium: 50 mg | Phosphorus: 60 mg | Potassium: 450 mg.

15 min | 15 min | 4

INGREDIENTS:

- One medium butternut squash peeled, seeded, and cut into half-inch cubes
- 2 tbsp olive oil
- 1 tbsp coconut sugar (or other natural sweeteners)
- 1 tsp ground cinnamon
- Salt to taste (keeping sodium below 20% of daily intake)

DIRECTIONS:

1. Mix butternut squash cubes with olive oil, coconut sugar, cinnamon, and a pinch of salt in a bowl.
2. Preheat the air fryer to 375°F (190°C).
3. Arrange the squash in the air fryer basket in a single layer and cook for 15 minutes, stirring halfway, until tender and golden.
4. Serve hot as a delightful side dish.

Heart-Healthy Benefits: *Dietary fiber and beta-carotene, abundant in butternut squash, can help maintain heart health. Coconut sugar provides a touch of sweetness with a lower glycemic index than regular sugar.*

NOTES

MEDITERRANEAN VEGETABLE MEDLEY

Calories: 90 kCal | Protein: 2 g | Carbohydrates: 11 g | Sugar: 6 g | Fat: 5 g | Fiber: 3 g | Cholesterol: 0 mg | Sodium: 60 mg | Phosphorus: 50 mg | Potassium: 340 mg.

15 min | 12 min | 4

INGREDIENTS:

- One zucchini, sliced into half-moons
- One bell pepper (any color), diced
- 1 cup cherry tomatoes, halved
- One red onion, diced
- 2 tbsp olive oil
- 1 tsp dried oregano
- Salt to taste (keeping sodium below 20% of daily intake)
- Freshly ground black pepper
- 2 tbsp fresh basil, chopped (for garnish)
- 2 tbsp vegan feta cheese (optional)

DIRECTIONS:

1. Combine zucchini, bell pepper, cherry tomatoes, and red onion in a large mixing bowl. Add olive oil, oregano, salt, and pepper, and toss well.
2. Preheat the air fryer to 380°F (190°C).
3. Transfer the vegetable mixture to the air fryer basket and cook for 12 minutes, shaking the basket halfway through until the veggies are tender.
4. Before serving, sprinkle with fresh basil and optional vegan feta cheese.

Heart-Healthy Benefits: *Zucchini and bell peppers are low in fat and high in dietary fiber, contributing to heart health. Tomatoes offer antioxidants like lycopene, which may reduce LDL cholesterol. Olive oil is a heart-friendly fat known to lower harmful cholesterol levels.*

SPICY PINEAPPLE CHICKEN WINGS

Calories: 180 kCal | Protein: 16 g | Carbohydrates: 12 g | Sugar: 10 g | Fat: 5 g | Fiber: 0,5 g | Cholesterol: 50 mg | Sodium: 230 mg | Phosphorus: 150 mg | Potassium: 250 mg.

10 min | 25 min | 4

INGREDIENTS:

- 1 lb chicken wings (skinless)
- 1/2 cup pineapple juice
- 2 tbsp soy sauce (low sodium)
- 1 tbsp honey
- 1 tsp chili flakes (adjust to taste)
- One garlic clove, minced
- Two green onions, sliced, for garnish

DIRECTIONS:

1. Mix pineapple juice, soy sauce, honey, chili flakes, and garlic in a bowl to create the marinade.
2. Add chicken wings to the bowl, ensuring they're coated well. Marinate for at least 30 minutes.
3. Preheat the air fryer to 380°F (193°C).
4. Remove chicken wings from the marinade and place them in a single layer in the air fryer basket. Cook for 25 minutes, turning halfway, until golden brown.
5. Garnish with green onions before serving.

Heart-Healthy Benefits: *Chicken, especially when skinless, is a lean source of protein. Pineapple juice provides bromelain, which may have anti-inflammatory properties beneficial for the heart. Soy sauce, used in moderation, offers a depth of flavor without excessive sodium.*

NOTES

TOMATO & MOZZARELLA CAPRESE SKEWERS

Calories: 110 kCal | Protein: 2 g | Carbohydrates: 8 g | Sugar: 5 g | Fat: 7 g | Fiber: 2 g | Cholesterol: 0 mg | Sodium: 50 mg | Phosphorus: 40 mg | Potassium: 250 mg.

15 min | 0 min | 4

INGREDIENTS:

- 1 pint cherry tomatoes
- 1 cup vegan mozzarella balls (or small cubes)
- 1/4 cup fresh basil leaves
- Olive oil for drizzling
- Balsamic glaze for drizzling
- Salt to taste (keeping sodium below 20% of daily intake)
- Freshly ground black pepper

DIRECTIONS:

1. Skewer a cherry tomato, a basil leaf, and a vegan mozzarella ball onto small skewers or toothpicks. Repeat with remaining ingredients.
2. Arrange skewers on a platter.
3. Drizzle with olive oil and balsamic glaze. Season with salt and freshly ground black pepper.

Heart-Healthy Benefits: *Lycopene, an abundant antioxidant in tomatoes, may lower the risk of heart disease. Olive oil is a healthy monounsaturated fat, beneficial for heart health. The vegan mozzarella alternative cuts down on saturated fats commonly found in dairy.*

GREEK LEMON OREGANO CHICKEN THIGHS

Calories: 250 kCal | Protein: 23 g | Carbohydrates: 2 g | Sugar: 1 g | Fat: 17 g | Fiber: 0,5 g | Cholesterol: 90 mg | Sodium: 150 mg | Phosphorus: 250 mg | Potassium: 300 mg.

15 min | 20 min 4 (plus marinating time)

INGREDIENTS:

- Four skinless chicken thighs
- Juice of 2 lemons
- Three garlic cloves, minced
- 2 tsp dried oregano
- 1/4 cup olive oil
- Salt to taste (mind the sodium content)
- Freshly ground black pepper

DIRECTIONS:

1. Combine lemon juice, minced garlic, oregano, olive oil, salt, and black pepper in a bowl. Mix well.
2. Marinate the chicken thighs in this mixture for at least 2 hours or overnight in the refrigerator.
3. Preheat the air fryer to 375°F (190°C).
4. Place chicken thighs in the air fryer basket in a single layer. Cook for 20 minutes or until fully cooked, turning halfway.
5. Serve warm, garnished with fresh lemon slices and additional oregano if desired.

Heart-Healthy Benefits: *Lemon provides vitamin C, an antioxidant, and oregano has anti-inflammatory properties.*

NOTES

PECAN-CRUSTED TROUT

Calories: 290 kCal | Protein: 28 g | Carbohydrates: 4 g | Sugar: 1 g | Fat: 20 g | Fiber: 2 g | Cholesterol: 75 mg | Sodium: 90 mg | Phosphorus: 200 mg | Potassium: 450 mg.

15 min | 15 min | 4

INGREDIENTS:

- Four trout fillets
- 1 cup ground pecans
- 1 tsp smoked paprika
- 1/2 tsp black pepper
- 2 tbsp olive oil
- Zest of 1 lemon
- Salt to taste (ensure low sodium)

DIRECTIONS:

1. Combine ground pecans, smoked paprika, lemon zest, black pepper, and salt in a bowl.
2. Brush trout fillets with olive oil, then press them into the pecan mixture, ensuring they are well coated.
3. Preheat the air fryer to 400°F (200°C).
4. Place the coated trout fillets in the air fryer in a single layer. Cook for 15 minutes or until the crust is golden and the trout is cooked.
5. Serve immediately with lemon wedges on the side.

Heart-Healthy Benefits:
Fish like trout are a great source of heart-healthy omega-3 fatty acids. Pecans contain antioxidants and healthy fats; olive oil provides heart-healthy monounsaturated fats.

CHILI LIME CAULIFLOWER STEAKS

Calories: 95 kCal | Protein: 3 g | Carbohydrates: 8 g | Sugar: 3 g | Fat: 7 g | Fiber: 3 g | Cholesterol: 0 mg | Sodium: 120 mg | Phosphorus: 50 mg | Potassium: 300 mg.

10 min | 18 min | 4

INGREDIENTS:

- One large cauliflower cut into 1-inch thick steaks
- 2 tbsp olive oil
- Zest and juice of 1 lime
- 1 tsp chili powder
- Salt to taste (remember the sodium content)
- Fresh cilantro for garnish (optional)

DIRECTIONS:

1. Whisk together olive oil, zest, lime juice, chili powder, and salt in a small bowl.
2. Brush each cauliflower steak with the chili-lime mixture.
3. Preheat the air fryer to 375°F (190°C).
4. Place cauliflower steaks in the air fryer in a single layer and cook for 18 minutes, flipping halfway through until they are tender and slightly crispy.
5. Garnish with fresh cilantro and serve immediately.

Heart-Healthy Benefits:
A great source of fiber that supports heart health is cauliflower. Olive oil, rich in monounsaturated fats, has been shown to reduce the risk of heart disease. The lime provides vitamin C, a potent antioxidant.

AIR-FRIED MINI BLUEBERRY MUFFINS

Calories: 85 kCal | Protein: 2 g | Carbohydrates: 18 g | Sugar: 5 g | Fat: 0,5 g | Fiber: 2 g | Cholesterol: 0 mg | Sodium: 100 mg | Phosphorus: 60 mg | Potassium: 85 mg.

10 min | 18 min | 4

INGREDIENTS:

- 1 cup whole wheat flour
- 1/2 cup almond milk
- 1/3 cup fresh blueberries
- 2 tbsp maple syrup
- 1 tsp baking powder
- 1/4 tsp vanilla extract
- 1/4 tsp salt (ensure low sodium)

DIRECTIONS:

6. Combine whole wheat flour, baking powder, and salt in a mixing bowl.
7. Add almond milk, maple syrup, and vanilla extract and mix until combined. Fold in blueberries.
8. Preheat the air fryer to 350°F (175°C).
9. Spoon the batter into mini muffin cups or silicone molds. Place the molds into the air fryer basket.
10. Cook for 12 minutes or until a toothpick inserted into a muffin comes clean.
11. Allow muffins to cool slightly before serving.

Heart-Healthy Benefits:
Whole wheat flour provides beneficial fiber, which can help reduce harmful LDL cholesterol levels. Blueberries are packed with antioxidants, which are known for their heart-protective benefits.

60-DAY MEAL PLAN

WEEK 1: KICKSTART TO HEART HEALTH

	Breakfast	Lunch	Dinner	Snack	Beverage
Day 1	Morning Berry Bliss Smoothie (18) & Nutty Quinoa Breakfast Delight (25)	Avocado & Quinoa Power Salad (31) with Ginger Pear Cooler Juice (19)	Lemon Herb Grilled Chicken Breasts (52) with Herb-Infused Olive Oil Dip (41)	Cherry Almond Morning Muffins (30)	Mango & Chia Seed Refreshment (73)
Day 2	Tropical Heart Health Delight (18) & Morning Glory Oat Bowl (25)	Grilled Zucchini & Pine Nut Medley (31) with Blackberry Mint Freshness Juice (22)	Lemon Herb Baked Salmon (64) with Rosemary & Lemon Vinaigrette (42)	Herb Roasted Veggie & Couscous Combo (35)	Herbal Berry Infusion (71)
Day 3	Carrot-Orange Revive Juice (21) & Savory Veggie Breakfast Muffins (26)	Avocado & Quinoa Power Salad (31) with Kiwi & Spinach Wake-Up Smoothie (20)	Honey Mustard Glazed Chicken Thighs (53) with Creamy Avocado & Lime Sauce (42)	Warm Cinnamon Apple & Rye Toast (30)	Strawberry Basil Quencher (72)
Day 4	Morning Berry Bliss Smoothie (18) & Cinnamon Apple Barley Porridge (24)	Cool Cucumber & Tuna Salad Sandwich (33) with Pomegranate Beet Zinger Juice (20)	Spiced Pork & Vegetable Stir-fry (58) with Herb-Crusted Pork Loin Roast (57)	Sesame & Date Morning Energy Balls (29)	Green Tea & Ginger Cooler (71)
Day 5	Creamy Avocado and Spinach Smoothie (72) & Mediterranean Feta & Veggie Omelette (26)	Cool Cucumber & Tuna Salad Sandwich (33) with Ruby Red Grapefruit Detox Juice (19)	Mediterranean Chicken Skewers (53) with Herb-Steamed Mussels with Lemon Zest (64)	Tomato Basil Mozzarella Sticks (36)	Creamy Avocado and spinach Smoothie (72)
Day 6	Mango & Strawberry Sunrise Smoothie (19) & Almond Crunch Yogurt Parfait (25)	Grilled Eggplant & Tomato Ciabatta (34) with Cranberry Almond Crunch Smoothie (22)	Rosemary Garlic Beef Skewers (58) with Golden Lentil & Spinach Soup (43)	Breezy Banana & Peanut Butter Roll-Ups (28)	Mango & Chia Seed Refreshment (73)
Day 7	Sunrise Berry Buckwheat Pancakes (27) & Raspberry Chia Overnight Oats (23)	Balsamic Mushroom & Arugula Baguette (35) with Creamy Avocado & Spinach Smoothie (72)	Herb-Infused Vegetable Medley Stew (49) with Cilantro Lime Turkey Burgers (55)	Herb Roasted Veggie & Couscous Combo (35)	Refreshing Cucumber Mint Water (71)

ADJUSTING & CUSTOMIZING YOUR MEAL PLAN:

Our 60-day meal plan has been designed with your heart health in mind, incorporating low-sodium, low-fat, and nutrient-rich recipes. However, each individual has unique needs and preferences.

- Mix and Match: If a particular meal doesn't appeal to you, swap it with another from the list. Ensure you're getting a good balance of nutrients throughout the day.
- Watch Portions: It's not just what you eat, but how much. Ensure you're adhering to recommended serving sizes.
- Stay Hydrated: Water plays a vital role in heart health. Aim for 8 cups daily, but adjust based on your activity level and body size.
- Listen to Your Body: If you feel hungry between meals, opt for heart-healthy snacks like nuts, fruits, or whole grains.
- Consult a Nutritionist or Doctor: It's always a good idea to speak with a health professional before making significant changes, especially if you have health issues or diseases. cholesterol, is now understood to have a more minor effect than previously thought. It's crucial to limit saturated and trans fats to maintain healthy cholesterol levels.

WEEK 2: Nutrient-Packed Favorites

	Breakfast	Lunch	Dinner	Snack	Beverage
Day 8	Tropical Fruit & Nut Salad (27) & Vanilla Chia & Berry Pudding Pot (28)	Mushroom & Quinoa Stuffed Bell Peppers (38) with Whole Wheat Spaghetti with Basil Pesto (39)	Honey-Ginger Glazed Tilapia (64) with Herb-Infused Olive Oil Dip (41)	Chickpea & Cucumber Salad Bowl (36)	Strawberry Basil Quencher (72)
Day 9	Morning Muesli with Dried Fruits (29) & Mediterranean Feta & Veggie Omelette (26)	Warm Mushroom & Lentil Salad (32) with Kiwi & Spinach Wake-Up Smoothie (20)	Mustard Glazed Pork Chops (59) with Silky Butternut Squash Soup (44)	Honey Drizzled Strawberry & Almond Plate (37)	Refreshing Cucumber Mint Water (71)
Day 10	Vanilla Chia & Berry Pudding Pot (28) & Creamy Avocado & Spinach Smoothie (72)	Open-Faced Avocado & Radish Toastie (34) with Mango and Chia Seed Refreshment (73)	Spiced Maple Turkey Sausages (56) with Carrot Ginger Puree (43)	Roasted Be l Pepper Strips with Hummus (37)	Cooling Watermelon & Lime Slush (72)
Day 11	Morning Glory Oat Bowl (25) & Cherry Vanilla Protein Smoothie (22)	Open-Faced Avocado & Radish Toastie (34) with Creamy Avocado & Lime Sauce (42)	Garlic & Herb Baked Turkey Meatballs (55) with Tuscan White Bean & Spinach Stew (50)	Tangy Apple Slices with Peanut Spread (38)	Pomegranate Green Tea Fusion (73)
Day 12	Raspberry Chia Overnight Oats (23) & Pomegranate Green Tea Fusion (109)	Cool Cucumber & Tuna Salad Sandwich (33) with Herb Roasted Veggie & Couscous Combo (35)	Mediterranean Shrimp & Vegetable Skewers (66) with Creamy Asparagus & Chive Soup (48)	Tomato Basil Mozzarella Sticks (36)	Heart-healthy Cocoa with a Hint of Cinnamon (74
Day 13	Kiwi & Spinach Wake-Up Smoothie (20) & Savory Veggie Breakfast Muffins (26)	Grilled Eggplant & Tomato Ciabatta (34) with Ruby Red Grapefruit Detox Juice (19)	Sesame Ginger Chicken Lettuce Wraps (54) with Golden Lentil & Spinach Soup (43)	Morning Muesli with Dried Fruits (29)	Soothing Fennel & Apple Drink (74)
Day 14	Tropical Heart Health Delight (18) & Nutty Quinoa Breakfast Delight (25)	Warm Mushroom & Lentil Salad (32) with Blackberry Mint Freshness Juice (22)	Balsamic Glazed Rainbow Trout (68) with Carrot Ginger Puree (43)	Cherry Almond Morning Muffins (30)	Creamy Avocado and Spinach Smoothie (72)

Engage with Your Food

- Cooking as Meditation: The process of cooking can be therapeutic. Engage in each step, from chopping to tasting, to make cooking a mindful practice.
- Garden-Fresh: If space allows, grow your herbs and some vegetables. Freshly harvested produce is not only flavorful but also heart-healthy.
- Stay Hydrated: Drink ample water throughout the day. Add fresh fruit or herbs to your water for flavor without adding calories.
- Dine Mindfully: Set aside electronics during meals. Eat slowly, savoring each bite, to improve digestion and recognize when you're full.
- Celebrate Often: Every time you choose a heart-healthy option, celebrate that choice. Over time, these celebrations reinforce positive eating habits.

Your relationship with food is a lifelong one. Engaging with it positively heart-healthy ensures the relationship is fulfilling and long-lasting. May each meal bring joy, health, and longevity to your life!

WEEK 3: DIVE INTO DELICIOUSNESS

	Breakfast	Lunch	Dinner	Snack	Beverage
Day 15	Sunrise Berry Buckwheat Pancakes (27) & Cinnamon Apple Barley Porridge (24)	Grilled Zucchini & Pine Nut Medley (31) with Kiwi & Spinach Wake-Up Smoothie (20)	Mediterranean Chicken Skewers (53) with Turmeric Infused Potato Leek Soup (46)	Breezy Banana & Peanut Butter Roll-Ups (28)	Heart-Healthy Cocoa with a Hint of Cinnamon (74)
Day 16	Mango & Strawberry Sunrise Smoothie (19) & Almond Crunch Yogurt Parfait (25)	Cool Cucumber & Tuna Salad Sandwich (33) with Pomegranate Beet Zinger Juice (20)	Tender Beef Medallions with Herbed Butter (59) with Cilantro-Lime Grilled Prawns (64)	Herb Roasted Veggie & Couscous Combo (35)	Herbal Berry Infusion (71)
Day 17	Mango & Strawberry Sunrise Smoothie (19) & Morning Glory Oat Bowl (25)	Mushroom & Quinoa Stuffed Bell Peppers (33) with Creamy Avocado & Lime Sauce (42)	Beef Sirloin & Caramelized Onion Bites (61) with Silky Butternut Squash Soup (44)	Sesame & Date Morning Energy Balls (29)	Mango & Chia Seed Refreshment (73)
Day 18	Mango & Strawberry Sunrise Smoothie (19) & Mediterranean Feta & Veggie Omelette (26)	Avocado & Quinoa Power Salad (31) with Ginger Pear Cooler Juice (19)	Lemon Herb Grilled Chicken Breasts (52) with Roasted Cauliflower & Nutmeg Soup (47)	Tomato Basil Mozzarella Sticks (36)	Herbal Berry Infusion (71)
Day 19	Carrot-Orange Revive Juice (21) & Morning Glory Oat Bowl (25)	Cool Cucumber & Tuna Salad Sandwich (33) with Pomegranate Beet Zinger Juice (20)	Herb-Infused Vegetable Medley Stew (49) with Cilantro Lime Turkey Burgers (55)	Chickpea & Cucumber Salad Bowl (36)	Herbal Berry Infusion (71)
Day 20	Mango & Strawberry Sunrise Smoothie (19) & Raspberry Chia Overnight Oats (23)	Grilled Zucchini & Pine Nut Medley (31) with Cranberry Almond Crunch Smoothie (22)	Beef Tenderloin with Roasted Asparagus (60) with Fiery Tomato and quinoa Stew (51)	Roasted Bell Pepper Strips with Hummus (37)	Cooling Watermelon & Lime Slush (72)
Day 21	Morning Berry Bliss Smoothie (18) & Savory Veggie Breakfast Muffins (26)	Warm Mushroom & Lentil Salad (32) with Kiwi & Spinach Wake-Up Smoothie (20)	Asian Inspired Beef & Broccoli (61) with Golden Lentil & Spinach Soup (43)	Warm Cinnamon Apple & Rye Toast (30)	Strawberry Basil Quencher (72)

Adjusting & Customizing Your Meal Plan:

As with any diet plan, individual needs can vary. Here are some guidelines for adapting the program:

- Substitute Ingredients: If you're allergic or sensitive to an ingredient, switch it out for something similar.
- Mind the Portions: You might need to adjust portion sizes depending on your personal calorie needs.
- Listen to Your Body: The most important thing is to stay attuned to your body's feelings and adjust your diet accordingly.
- Keep It Varied: The provided plan aims to ensure nutritional adequacy and provide a variety of tastes. However, repeating meals or mixing and matching days is perfectly fine.

WEEK 4: SAVORY SENSATIONS

	Breakfast	Lunch	Dinner	Snack	Beverage
Day 22	Tropical Heart Health Delight (18) & Nutty Quinoa Breakfast Delight (25)	Grilled Eggplant & Tomato Ciabatta (34) with Mango & Chia Seed Refreshment (73)	Spiced Pork & Vegetable Stir-fry (58) with Herb-Steamed Mussels with Lemon Zest (64)	Honey Drizzled Strawberry & Almond Plate (37)	Cooling Watermelon & Lime Slush (72)
Day 23	Morning Berry Bliss Smoothie (18) & Morning Glory Oat Bowl (25)	Avocado & Quinoa Power Salad (31) with Creamy Avocado & Spinach Smoothie (72)	Garlic Butter Lobster Tails (65) with Roasted Red Beet and Dill Soup (45)	Breezy Banana & Peanut Butter Roll-Ups (28)	Herbal Berry Infusion (71)
Day 24	Cranberry Almond Crunch Smoothie (22) & Mediterranean Feta & Veggie Omelette (26)	Open-Faced Avocado & Radish Toastie (34) with Blackberry Mint Freshness Juice (22)	Herb-Infused Vegetable Medley Stew (49) with Garlic & Herb Baked Turkey Meatballs (55)	Chickpea & Cucumber Salad Bowl (36)	Soothing Fennel & Apple Drink (74)
Day 25	Tropical Fruit & Nut Salad (27) & Almond Crunch Yogurt Parfait (25)	Mushroom & Quinoa Stuffed Bell Peppers (38) with Cranberry Almond Crunch Smoothie (22)	Mint & Garlic Roasted Chicken Quarters (57) with Turmeric Infused Potato Leek Soup (46)	Herb Roasted Veggie & Couscous Combo (35)	Soothing Fennel & Apple Drink (74)
Day 26	Morning Muesli with Dried Fruits (29) & Sunrise Berry Buckwheat Pancakes (27)	Grilled Eggplant & Tomato Ciabatta (34) with Ginger Pear Cooler Juice (19)	Mustard Glazed Pork Chops (59) with Golden Lentil & Spinach Soup (43)	Cherry Almond Morning Muffins (30)	Soothing Fennel & Apple Drink (74)
Day 27	Kiwi & Spinach Wake-Up Smoothie (20) & Raspberry Chia Overnight Oats (23)	Cool Cucumber & Tuna Salad Sandwich (33) with Pomegranate Beet Zinger Juice (20)	Herb-crusted pork Loin Roast (51) with Silky Butternut Squash Soup (44)	Tomato Basil Mozzarella Sticks (36)	Herbal Berry Infusion (71)
Day 28	Mango & Strawberry Sunrise Smoothie (19) & Avocado and poached Egg Toast (24)	Grilled Eggplant & Tomato Ciabatta (34) with Cranberry Almond Crunch Smoothie (22)	Zesty Orange Baked Mackerel (68) with Tuscan White Bean and Spinach Stew (50)	Roasted Bell Pepper Strips with Hummus (37)	Creamy Avocado and spinach Smoothie (72)

Practical Cooking Tips

- Prepare in Advance: Consider preparing some meals or ingredients in advance, especially for busy days. This can help you avoid unhealthy last-minute choices.
- Use Fresh Herbs: Fresh herbs like basil, cilantro, and rosemary add flavor and have health benefits.
- Opt for Whole Grains: Whenever possible, choose whole grains like brown rice, quinoa, and whole wheat pasta. They're more nutritious and filling.
- Watch the Oils: Use heart-healthy oils like olive or avocado oil for cooking. However, use them sparingly as they're calorie-dense.
- Steam or Grill: Steaming and grilling are excellent methods to retain food nutrients. Plus, they add minimal fats.
- Store Properly: Store fruits and vegetables in appropriate conditions to maintain their freshness and nutritional value.

WEEK 5: FLAVORFUL FEAST

	Breakfast	Lunch	Dinner	Snack	Beverage
Day 29	Carrot-Orange Revive Juice (21) & Savory Veggie Breakfast Muffins (26)	Warm Mushroom & Lentil Salad (32) with Kiwi & Spinach Wake-Up Smoothie (20)	Mediterranean Chicken Skewers (53) with Spinach and Feta Cream Soup (47)	Honey Drizzled Strawberry & Almond Plate (37)	Strawberry Basil Quencher (72)
Day 30	Morning Berry Bliss Smoothie (18) & Morning Glory Oat Bowl (25)	Grilled Zucchini & Pine Nut Medley (31) with Ginger Pear Cooler Juice (19)	Rosemary Infused Turkey Tenderloin (57) with Herb-Infused Olive Oil Dip (41)	Warm Cinnamon Apple & Rye Toast (30)	Green Tea & Ginger Cooler (71)
Day 31	Tropical Heart Health Delight (18) & Almond Crunch Yogurt Parfait (25)	Avocado & Quinoa Power Salad (31) with Pomegranate Beet Zinger Juice (20)	Herb-crusted pork Loin Roast (57) with Spiced Chickpea and Spinach Stew (49)	Cherry Almond Morning Muffins (30)	Heart-healthy Cocoa with a Hint of Cinnamon (74)
Day 32	Creamy Avocado and Spinach Smoothie (72) & Nutty Quinoa Breakfast Delight (25)	Grilled Eggplant & Tomato Ciabatta (34) with Mango & Strawberry Sunrise Smoothie (19)	Basil & Tomato Shrimp Bruschetta (66) with Golden Lentil & Spinach Soup (43)	Sesame & Date Morning Energy Balls (29)	Herbal Berry Infusion (71)
Day 33	Cherry Vanilla Protein Smoothie (22) & Mediterranean Feta & Veggie Omelette (26)	Cool Cucumber and Tuna Salad Sandwich (33) with Creamy Avocado and spinach Smoothie (72)	Beef & Bell Pepper Kebabs (53) with Sweet Corn & Bell Pepper Chowder (44)	Tomato Basil Mozzarella Sticks (36)	Green Tea & Ginger Cooler (71)
Day 34	Carrot-Orange Revive Juice (21) & Mediterranean Feta & Veggie Omelette (26)	Grilled Zucchini & Pine Nut Medley (31) with Blackberry Mint Freshness Juice (22)	Cilantro Lime Turkey Burgers (55) with Hearty Beet & Carrot Stew (51)	Roasted Bell Pepper Strips with Hummus (37)	Soothing Fennel & Apple Drink (74)
Day 35	Kiwi & Spinach Wake-Up Smoothie (20) & Morning Glory Oat Bowl (25)	Mushroom & Quinoa Stuffed Bell Peppers (38) with Creamy Avocado & Lime Sauce (42)	Tuscan Herb Grilled Sardines (68) with Roasted Red Beet and Dill Soup (45)	Breezy Banana & Peanut Butter Roll-Ups (28)	Pomegranate Green Tea Fusion (73)

TIPS FOR ADAPTING THE MEAL GUIDE:

- Your Body: If you're still hungry after a meal, add more vegetables or a serving of lean protein.
- Substitute Wisely: If you dislike an ingredient, replace it with something you prefer, but always ensure it aligns with the heart-healthy goals.
- Meal Prep: Some of these dishes can be prepared beforehand, making it easier for those with a busy lifestyle.
- Keep an Eye on Portions: While these recipes are heart-healthy, portion control is essential.
- Stay Hydrated: Drink a lot of water all day long. You can also enjoy beverages like the Herbal Berry Infusion or Green Tea & Ginger Cooler.

Remember, while this meal plan is structured, it's not set in stone. Use it as a guideline, and feel free to mix and match recipes based on what you have available and what you're in the mood for. Healthy eating is about balance, variety, and listening to your body. Enjoy your culinary journey to a healthier heart!

WEEK 6: HEALTHY HARMONY

	Breakfast	Lunch	Dinner	Snack	Beverage
Day 36	Tropical Fruit & Nut Salad (27) & Raspberry Chia Overnight Oats (23)	Avocado and radish Toastie (34) with Pomegranate Beet Zinger Juice (20)	Mediterranean Chicken Skewers (53) with Shrimp & Avocado Lettuce Wraps (65)	Morning Muesli with Dried Fruits (29)	Strawberry Basil Quencher (72)
Day 37	Mango & Strawberry Sunrise Smoothie (19) & Savory Veggie Breakfast Muffins (26)	Grilled Zucchini & Pine Nut Medley (31) with Ginger Pear Cooler Juice (19)	Mustard Glazed Pork Chops (59) with Roasted Cauliflower & Nutmeg Soup (47)	Chickpea & Cucumber Salad Bowl (36)	Mango & Chia Seed Refreshment (73)
Day 38	Morning Berry Bliss Smoothie (18) & Nutty Quinoa Breakfast Delight (23)	Open-Faced Avocado & Radish Toastie (34) with Cranberry Almond Crunch Smoothie (22)	Lemon Herb Grilled Chicken Breasts (52) with Creamy Asparagus & Chive Soup (48)	Herb Roasted Veggie & Couscous Combo (35)	Herbal Berry Infusion (71)
Day 39	Tropical Heart Health Delight (18) & Raspberry Chia Overnight Oats (23)	Warm Mushroom and lentil Salad (32) with Creamy Avocado and Spinach Smoothie (72)	Beef Sirloin & Caramelized Onion Bites (61) with Herb-Infused Vegetable Medley Stew (49)	Tomato Basil Mozzarella Sticks (36)	Cooling Watermelon & Lime Slush (72)
Day 40	Mango & Strawberry Sunrise Smoothie (19) & Mediterranean Feta & Veggie Omelette (26)	Grilled Eggplant & Tomato Ciabatta (34) with Cranberry Almond Crunch Smoothie (22)	Tuscan Herb Chicken & Vegetable Roast (56) with Golden Lentil & Spinach Soup (43)	Roasted Bell Pepper Strips with Hummus (37)	Soothing Fennel & Apple Drink (74)
Day 41	Morning Berry Bliss Smoothie (18) & Almond Crunch Yogurt Parfait (25)	Cool Cucumber & Tuna Salad Sandwich (33) with Pomegranate Beet Zinger Juice (20)	Beef & Mushroom Stuffed Tomatoes (63) with Tuscan White Bean & Spinach Stew (50)	Sesame & Date Morning Energy Balls (29)	Strawberry Basil Quencher (72)
Day 42	Kiwi & Spinach Wake-Up Smoothie (20) & Nutty Quinoa Breakfast Delight (25)	Avocado and radish Toastie (34) with Cranberry Almond Crunch Smoothie (22)	Thyme & Lemon Grilled Grouper (69) with Silky Butternut Squash Soup (44)	Cherry Almond Morning Muffins (30)	Heart-healthy Cocoa with a Hint of Cinnamon (74)

EMBRACE LIFE'S UPS AND DOWN

- Stay Adaptable: Life is unpredictable. Flexibility is vital to maintaining a balanced lifestyle. When things don't go as planned, don't stress. Adapt and move forward.
- Practice Self-Compassion: Be gentle with yourself. Celebrate your achievements, no matter how small, and learn from your mistakes without harsh self-judgment.
- Reconnect: Spend quality time with loved ones or indulge in hobbies that make you happy. These moments can act as a reset button during hectic times.
- Plan but Let Go: A plan is beneficial, but sometimes things don't align. When this happens, let go and trust the journey.

WEEK 7: Nutritious Novelties

	Breakfast	Lunch	Dinner	Snack	Beverage
Day 43	Tropical Fruit & Nut Salad (27) & Morning Glory Oat Bowl (25)	Broccoli & Cauliflower in Lemon Vinaigrette (39) with Ginger Pear Cooler Juice (19)	Mediterranean Chicken Skewers (53) with Cool Cucumber & Avocado Gazpacho (45)	Morning Muesli with Dried Fruits (29)	Green Tea & Ginger Cooler (71)
Day 44	Mango & Strawberry Sunrise Smoothie (19) & Savory Veggie Breakfast Muffins (26)	Grilled Eggplant & Tomato Ciabatta (34) with Blackberry Mint Freshness Juice (22)	Herb-Infused Vegetable Medley Stew (49) with Garlic & Herb Baked Turkey Meatballs (55)	Herb Roasted Veggie & Couscous Combo (35)	Cooling Watermelon & Lime Slush (72)
Day 45	Carrot-Orange Revive Juice (21) & Savory Veggie Breakfast Muffins (26)	Warm Mushroom & Lentil Salad (32) with Creamy Avocado & Spinach Smoothie (72)	Rosemary Infused Turkey Tenderloin (52) with Spinach & Feta Cream Soup (47)	Honey Drizzled Strawberry & Almond Plate (37)	Herbal Berry Infusion (71)
Day 46	Mango & Strawberry Sunrise Smoothie (19) & Savory Veggie Breakfast Muffins (26)	Avocado & Quinoa Power Salad (31) with Morning Berry Bliss Smoothie (18)	Savory Herb Pork Ribs (Slow-Cooked) (60) with Hearty Mushroom and pearl Barley Stew (50)	Roasted Bell Pepper Strips with Hummus (37)	Herbal Berry Infusion (71)
Day 47	Mango & Strawberry Sunrise Smoothie (19) & Mediterranean Feta & Veggie Omelette (26)	Grilled Eggplant & Tomato Ciabatta (34) with Pomegranate Beet Zinger Juice (20)	Cumin Lime Pork Steaks (62) with Silky Butternut Squash Soup (44)	Sesame & Date Morning Energy Balls (29)	Green Tea & Ginger Cooler (71)
Day 48	Carrot-Orange Revive Juice (21) & Almond Crunch Yogurt Parfait (25)	Warm Mushroom & Lentil Salad (32) with Creamy Avocado and spinach Smoothie (72)	Rosemary Infused Baked Pollock (69) with Hearty Beet & Carrot Stew (51)	Tomato Basil Mozzarella Sticks (36)	Strawberry Basil Quencher (72)
Day 49	Kiwi & Spinach Wake-Up Smoothie (20) & Morning Glory Oat Bowl (25)	Mushroom & Quinoa Stuffed Bell Peppers (38) with Ginger Pear Cooler Juice (19)	Honey Mustard Glazed Chicken Thighs (53) with Creamy Asparagus & Chive Soup (48)	Morning Muesli with Dried Fruits (29)	Cooling Watermelon & Lime Slush (72)

Dietary Notes & Guidance

- Balance is Key: While these meals are crafted for heart health, ensuring you receive a comprehensive range of nutrients is essential. Consider incorporating a variety of fruits and vegetables to get the full spectrum of vitamins and minerals.
- Mindful Eating: Be present during meals. Eating slowly and savoring each bite can aid digestion and help you recognize when you're full.
- Limit Processed Foods: While they may be convenient, processed foods often contain added sugars, unhealthy fats, and high sodium levels. Opt for fresh ingredients whenever possible.
- Consider Supplements: If you have specific health concerns or feel you're not getting certain nutrients, consult a healthcare provider about possibly adding supplements to your routine.
- Stay Active: A heart-healthy diet is most effective with regular exercise. Aim for 150 minutes or more per week of aerobic exercise at a moderate level.
- Regular Checkups: Visit your healthcare provider regularly to monitor cholesterol, blood pressure, and other heart-related metrics.

WEEK 8: Wholesome Wrap-Up

	Breakfast	Lunch	Dinner	Snack	Beverage
Day 50	Tropical Heart Health Delight (18) & Morning Glory Oat Bowl (25)	Grilled Zucchini & Pine Nut Medley (31) with Cranberry Almond Crunch Smoothie (22)	Mediterranean Chicken Skewers (53) with Herb-Infused Vegetable Medley Stew (49)	Cherry Almond Morning Muffins (30)	Soothing Fennel & Apple Drink (74)
Day 51	Mango & Strawberry Sunrise Smoothie (19) & Raspberry Chia Overnight Oats (23)	Grilled Zucchini & Pine Nut Medley (31) with Kiwi & Spinach Wake-Up Smoothie (20)	Lemon Herb Grilled Chicken Breasts (52) with Golden Lentil & Spinach Soup (43)	Breezy Banana & Peanut Butter Roll-Ups (28)	Celery & Apple Cleanse Juice (74)
Day 52	Morning Berry Bliss Smoothie (18) & Nutty Quinoa Breakfast Delight (25)	Open-Faced Avocado & Radish Toastie (34) with Pomegranate Beet Zinger Juice (20)	Rosemary Garlic Beef Skewers (58) with Silky Butternut Squash Soup (44)	Open-Faced Avocado & Radish Toastie (34)	Green Tea & Ginger Cooler (71)
Day 53	Tropical Fruit & Nut Salad (27) & Mediterranean Feta & Veggie Omelette (26)	Cool Cucumber & Tuna Salad Sandwich (33) with Blackberry Mint Freshness Juice (22)	Savory Herb Pork Ribs (Slow-Cooked) (60) with Creamy Asparagus & Chive Soup (48)	Sesame & Date Morning Energy Balls (29)	Creamy Avocado & Spinach Smoothie (72)
Day 54	Mango & Strawberry Sunrise Smoothie (19) & Raspberry Chia Overnight Oats (23)	Grilled Eggplant & Tomato Ciabatta (34) with Ginger Pear Cooler Juice (19)	Lemon Butter Seared Salmon Fillets (70) with Sweet Corn and bell Pepper Chowder (44)	Roasted Bell Pepper Strips with Hummus (37)	Green Tea & Ginger Cooler (71)
Day 55	Morning Berry Bliss Smoothie (18) & Savory Veggie Breakfast Muffins (26)	Mushroom & Quinoa Stuffed Bell Peppers (38) with Creamy Avocado & Spinach Smoothie (72)	Shrimp & Avocado Lettuce Wraps (65) with Creamy Asparagus & Chive Soup (48)	Honey Drizzled Strawberry & Almond Plate (37)	Herbal Berry Infusion (71)
Day 56	Kiwi & Spinach Wake-Up Smoothie (20) & Morning Glory Oat Bowl (25)	Warm Mushroom & Lentil Salad (32) with Pomegranate Beet Zinger Juice (20)	Soy-Ginger Glazed Pork Skewers (62) with Golden Lentil & Spinach Soup (43)	Cherry Almond Morning Muffins (30)	Strawberry Basil Quencher (72)

Further Dietary Recommendations

- Snacking Wisely: Opt for snacks that are high in fiber and protein. This will satisfy your hunger and stabilize your blood sugar levels.
- Avoid Excessive Caffeine: While a cup or two of coffee can be beneficial, excessive caffeine can lead to high blood pressure. Opt for herbal teas or decaffeinated versions if needed.
- Limit Alcohol Intake: Alcohol can raise blood pressure and add extra calories. If consumed, do so in moderation.
- Stay Informed: Continually educate yourself about heart-healthy foods and keep abreast of new research. This will empower you to make the best decisions for your heart health.
- Incorporate Omega-3 Fatty Acids: Foods like salmon, flaxseed, and walnuts are rich in omega-3s, which are beneficial for heart health.
- Keep Stress at Bay: Chronic stress can negatively impact heart health. Incorporate relaxation techniques like meditation, deep breathing, and gentle exercise into your daily routine.

Remember, a heart-healthy lifestyle isn't just about the foods you eat. It's also about maintaining a balanced lifestyle that includes regular exercise, adequate sleep, and emotional well-being. Embrace this holistic approach for optimal heart health and overall well-being.

WEEK 9: CULINARY CONCLUSIONS

	Breakfast	Lunch	Dinner	Snack	Beverage
Day 57	Tropical Heart Health Delight (18) & Mediterranean Feta & Veggie Omelette (26)	Avocado & Quinoa Power Salad (31) with Cranberry Almond Crunch Smoothie (22)	Herb-Crusted Pork Loin Roast (57) with Tuscan White Bean & Spinach Stew (50)	Tomato Basil Mozzarella Sticks (36)	Pomegranate Green Tea Fusion (73)
Day 58	Mango & Strawberry Sunrise Smoothie (19) & Nutty Quinoa Breakfast Delight (25)	Grilled Zucchini & Pine Nut Medley (31)	Tuscan Herb Chicken & Vegetable Roast (56) with Creamy Asparagus & Chive Soup (48)	Herb Roasted Veggie & Couscous Combo (35)	Cooling Watermelon & Lime Slush (72)
Day 59	Carrot-Orange Revive Juice (21) & Savory Veggie Breakfast Muffins (26)	Warm Mushroom & Lentil Salad (32) with Creamy Avocado and Spinach Smoothie (72)	Lemon Herb Grilled Chicken Breasts (52) with Tuscan White Bean & Spinach Stew (50)	Morning Muesli with Dried Fruits (29)	Green Tea & Ginger Cooler (71)
Day 60	Cherry Vanilla Protein Smoothie (22) & Almond Crunch Yogurt Parfait (25)	Broccoli & Cauliflower in Lemon Vinaigrette (39) with Ginger Pear Cooler Juice (19)	Cumin & Lime Baked Catfish (70) with Silky Butternut Squash Soup (44)	Roasted Bell Pepper Strips with Hummus (37)	Heart-healthy Cocoa with a Hint of Cinnamon (74)
Day 61	Tropical Fruit & Nut Salad (27) & Mediterranean Feta & Veggie Omelette (26)	Grilled Eggplant & Tomato Ciabatta (34) with Blackberry Mint Freshness Juice (22)	Mediterranean Chicken Skewers (53) with Hearty Potato & Green Onion Soup (48)	Sesame & Date Morning Energy Balls (29)	Cooling Watermelon & Lime Slush (72)
Day 62	Creamy Avocado and Spinach Smoothie (72) & Morning Glory Oat Bowl (25)	Avocado & Quinoa Power Salad (31) with Pomegranate Beet Zinger Juice (20)	Tarragon & Orange Roasted Chicken (54) with Tuscan White Bean & Spinach Stew (50)	Cherry Almond Morning Muffins (30)	Heart-healthy Cocoa with a Hint of Cinnamon (74)
Day 63	Morning Berry Bliss Smoothie (18) & Nutty Quinoa Breakfast Delight (25)	Warm Mushroom and lentil Salad (32) with Creamy Avocado and Spinach Smoothie (72)	Beef & Mushroom Stuffed Tomatoes (63) with Spiced Chickpea & Spinach Stew (49)	Tomato Basil Mozzarella Sticks (36)	Green Tea & Ginger Cooler (71)

BEYOND THE PLATE: EMBRACING A HOLISTIC LIFESTYLE

- Physical Activity: Integrate cardiovascular exercises like walking, swimming, or cycling, which can help keep the heart strong and improve circulation.
- Mental Health: Regular meditation, relaxation exercises, or even simple deep-breathing techniques can reduce stress, a significant factor affecting heart health.
- Limiting Toxins: Reduce or eliminate the intake of tobacco and excessive alcohol, as these can harm heart health.
- Regular Checkups: Besides self-monitoring, visit healthcare professionals for routine checks to ensure cholesterol, blood pressure, and other vital metrics are checked.
- Sleep: Ensure you get 7-9 hours; rest is essential for heart health and overall well-being.

As our 63-day journey concludes, reflecting on the newfound culinary experiences and the positive impact on heart health is essential. The real success comes from integrating these dietary habits into one's daily life long-term, allowing for a foundation of health and well-being. Repeating some of these recipes, alternating them, or introducing new heart-healthy recipes can help maintain this lifestyle beyond the 63 days. Remember, ongoing consultation with nutritionists or dieticians can provide guidance tailored to individual needs and preferences.

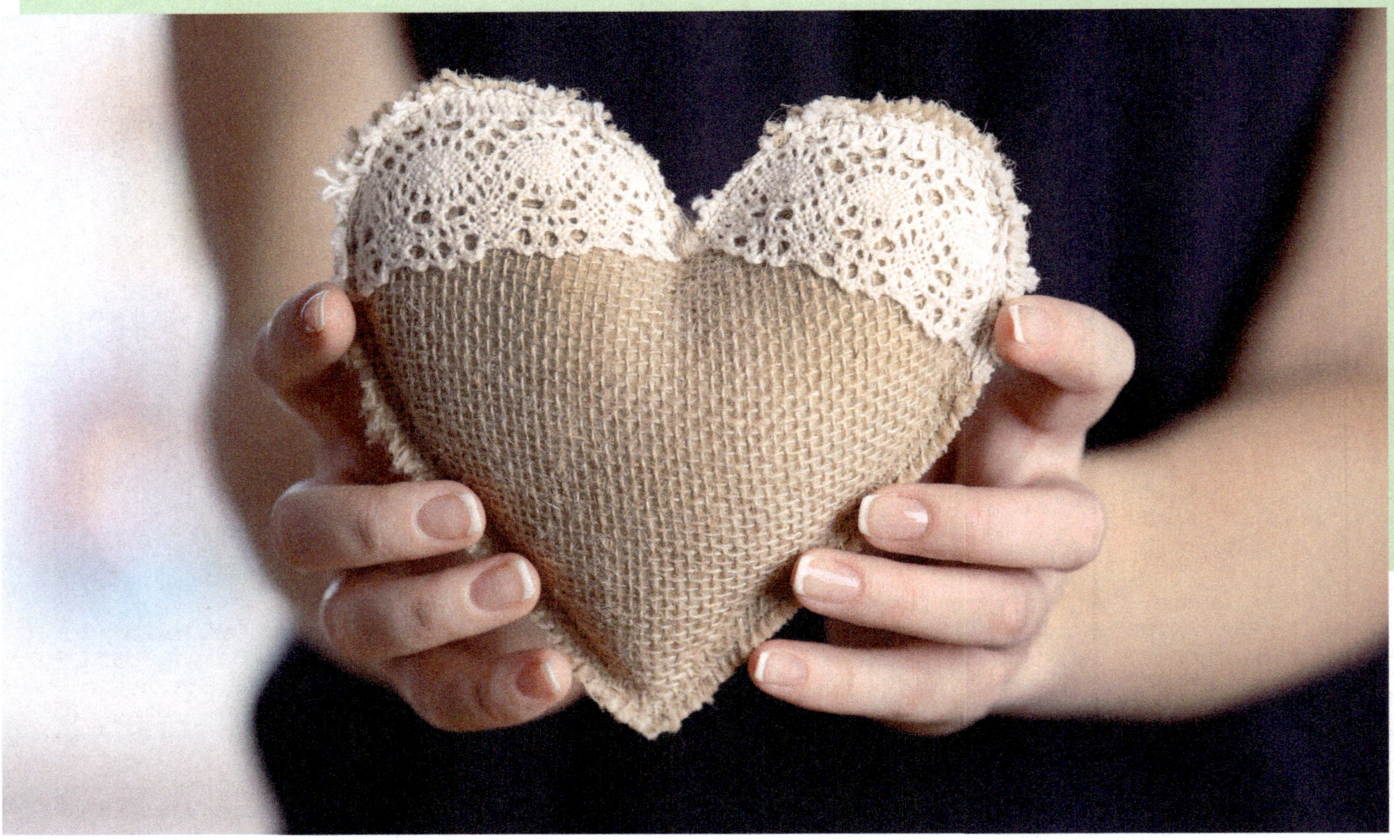

Insights from the Experts

Current Research & Findings on Heart Health

Modern medicine and nutrition science are ever-evolving fields. Constant research yields discoveries, offering more profound insights into heart health and how our dietary and lifestyle choices impact it. Here are some of the latest findings:

- Link Between Gut Health and Heart Health: Recent studies have illuminated the intricate connection between our gut microbiome and heart health. A balanced gut can reduce inflammation, a significant contributor to cardiovascular diseases. Consuming a fiber-rich diet and fermented foods can support a healthy microbiome.
- Plant Sterols & Heart Health: Foods fortified with plant sterols or naturally containing them have reduced harmful LDL cholesterol levels. These compounds in certain plants block cholesterol from being absorbed into the bloodstream.
- Reduced Red Meat Consumption: A meta-analysis of various research studies indicates that replacing red meat with plant-based proteins, like legumes and nuts, can significantly reduce heart disease risk factors.
- Importance of Sleep: Heart health is not just about diet and exercise. Recent research emphasizes the critical role of sleep. Chronic sleep deprivation can lead to problems like obesity, high blood pressure, and even heart attacks.

Tips for Sustaining a Heart-Healthy Diet Long-Term

A heart-healthy diet is not a short-term fix but a lifelong commitment. Here are expert tips to make this journey sustainable and enjoyable:

- Stay Updated: With new research emerging regularly, it's beneficial to stay updated. This could mean subscribing to health newsletters, joining a health community, or routinely visiting your nutritionist.
- Variety is Key: Introduce a variety of foods in your diet. This ensures you get a spectrum of nutrients and prevents mealtime monotony.
- Plan Ahead: Whether it's meal prepping for the week, having a list for grocery shopping, or knowing heart-healthy restaurants nearby, planning can help you avoid last-minute unhealthy choices.
- Share the Journey: Involve family and friends. When the entire household adopts a heart-healthy lifestyle, it becomes more manageable and fun. Plus, sharing recipes and tips can be exceptionally motivating.
- Mindful Eating: Pay attention to what you eat. Listen to your body. Recognize when you're hungry and when you're satiated. Mindful eating can prevent overeating and improve digestion.
- Revisit and Reflect: Set aside time every month or quarter to reflect on your heart-healthy journey. Celebrate the victories, no matter how small, and adjust where necessary.
- Incorporating the latest findings on heart health into our lives can seem daunting initially. Still, with determination and a genuine understanding of the benefits, it becomes an integral part of our lifestyle. These expert tips ensure that your heart-healthy journey is not just a phase but a lasting change, promoting a lifetime of robust heart health.

Conclusion: Embracing a Lifelong Commitment to Heart Health

As we end our heart-healthy exploration together, it's imperative to underscore a pivotal understanding: the journey to heart health is neither a temporary phase nor a fleeting trend. Instead, it's an enduring commitment, a vow we make to our hearts and, by extension, to ourselves.

Throughout this book, we've traversed the vast landscape of heart-healthy eating. We've equipped ourselves with knowledge, recipes, and expert insights. But this is merely the start. To truly cherish the benefits, we must weave these principles into the very fabric of our daily lives.

Why This Commitment Matters

Your heart, a marvelous organ, pumps tirelessly from the moment you're born until your last breath. It asks for so little in return: just a bit of care, mindfulness, and nourishment. By prioritizing heart health, you're elongating your life and amplifying its quality. A healthy heart translates to increased vitality, better stamina, and a heightened capacity to relish life's simple pleasures.

The Lifelong Journey

As with any journey, there will be moments of triumph and stumbling. Some days, you indulge more than you planned or skip your exercise. That's alright. Perfection isn't the goal here; consistency is. It's about getting back on track, reminding yourself of why this journey began in the first place, and moving forward with renewed vigor.

Support Systems

Lean on your community — be it family, friends, or online groups dedicated to heart health. Share your milestones, seek advice during challenging times, and continually educate yourself. This community will be your anchor, offering encouragement when the path seems daunting.

Continuous Learning

The realm of health and nutrition is ever-evolving. New studies emerge, offering fresh insights. Stay curious. Be open to adapting and fine-tuning your approach based on the latest knowledge. This adaptability ensures that your heart-healthy regimen remains both relevant and practical.

The Heart's Gratitude

Your heart notices every wholesome meal you consume, every active choice you make. And in its unique, silent way, it thanks you. The steady, rhythmic beats, the absence of ailments, and the sheer energy you feel are your heart's tokens of gratitude.

In closing, embracing a heart-healthy lifestyle is among the most profound gifts you can bestow upon yourself. It's a declaration of self-love, self-respect, and a desire to live fully. As you stand at this pivotal juncture, ready to embark on or continue this heart-healthy journey, know that every positive choice you make echoes in the harmonious beats of your grateful heart.

Here's to a life brimming with heart-driven adventures and healthful moments. To the heart that beats within you and the choices that keep it thriving — Cheers!

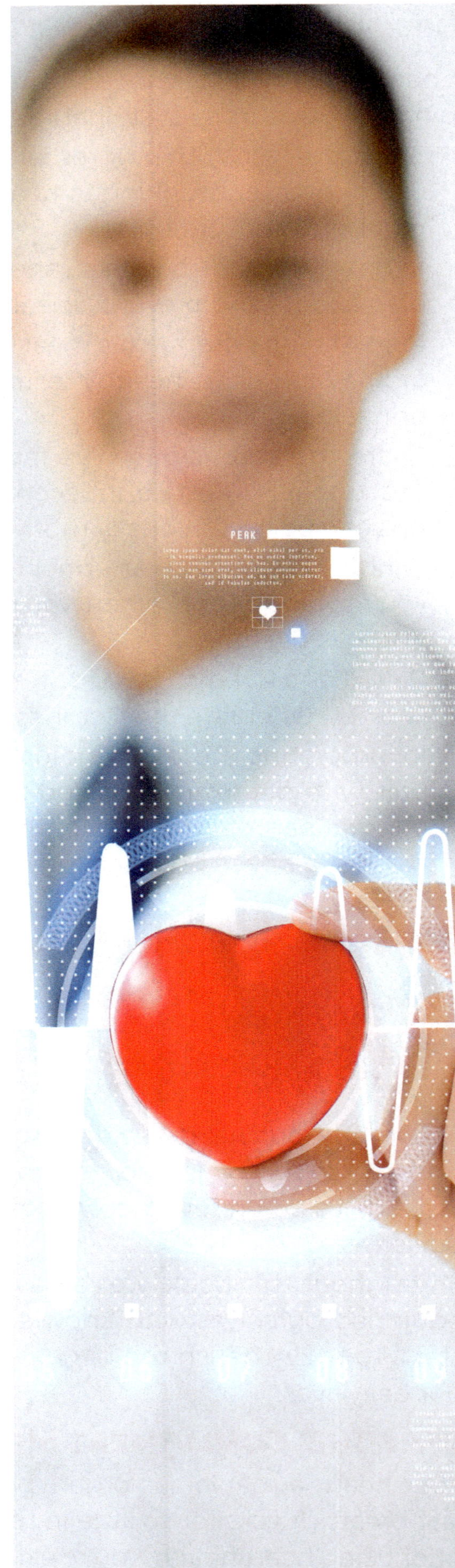

Printed in Great Britain
by Amazon

42571904R00057